W9-ARK-278

MENTAL HEALTH NURSING MANUAL

Second Edition

NORMA S. DE CASTRO, R.N., PH.D.

Humber College of Applied Arts and Technology
Health Sciences Division
Nursing Department
Rexdale, Ontario, Canada

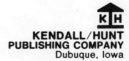

KENDALL/HUNT PUBLISHING COMPANY
Dubuque, Iowa

TO MY STUDENTS,
WHO ARE THE BEST TEACHERS
FOR THEY TAUGHT ME TO BE
A STUDENT OF MY OWN TEACHING

–Norma S. de Castro

Formerly entitled *Mental Health Nursing Workbook*

Copyright © 1983, 1984 by Kendall/Hunt Publishing Company

ISBN 0-8403-3269-6

All rights reserved. No part of this publication may be reproduced, stored in a retrieval system, or transmitted, in any form or by any means, electronic, mechanical, photocopying, recording, or otherwise, without the prior written permission of the copyright owner.

Printed in the United States of America

B   403269   01

Contents

Suggested Learning Activities

Preface to the Second Edition

The initial impetus to write the first edition of Mental Health Nursing Workbook began with the compilation of learning activities while teaching student nurses in their Psychiatric-Mental Health nursing studies and conducting workshops and seminars to many different groups in the health professions. Preface to the first edition reads "Much of what happened in psychiatric nursing before is now being recognized as a significant aspect of all nursing and is applicable to any given setting. This transformation poses a set of dilemmas to learners who are just beginning their psychiatric nursing experience as the skills learned in this area are not only for clients with emotional and mental problems but extend to all areas of nursing practice. It is not uncommon to hear learners state 'we wish we had the experience before we began to nurse in other areas' ".

The Mental Health Nursing Workbook is now revised into a manual in response to positive comments both from learners and colleagues from all over Canada and the United States and to reflect the author's continuing interest in making psychiatric-mental health nursing understandable to the learner. Learning at the best of times is not an easy process and this is not made any easier by the proliferation and availability of textbooks in the area. Every attempt has been made to limit detail and elaboration beyond the basic clinical aspect and to concentrate instead on the essential features of acquiring a working knowledge of a particular subject that is related to nurses' role.

The purpose and character of the manual remain what they were, as a workbook, but the subjects have been expanded, elaborated and presented in easily understandable terms, taking only a few liberties with theory and details as necessary to maintain simplicity. Many authors of psychiatric nursing textbooks will find that their concepts and conclusions are utilized and adapted to the scheme of the presentation.

Suggested readings at the end of each chapter have been carefully chosen both for usefulness and to introduce the learners to the wide range of textbooks available, to research details and facts.

Learning activities are provided at the conclusion of each section to stimulate learning through experiential modes rather than to suggest specific answers to problems of maladaptation.

The value of the manual lies not so much in the range of its content as in the choice and simplicity of the specific subjects which it contains to increase better understanding and appreciation of psychiatric-mental health nursing, both for learners who are just beginning their nursing studies and for those nurses working in psychiatric community agencies who wish to update their nursing skills.

The author is hopeful that at the conclusion of the study, the learner will:

– be effective in his or her client interaction

– will establish a therapeutic nurse-client relationship

– gain insight into own behavior

– practice and utilize therapeutic communication techniques

– participate in psychosocial assessment

– develop skills in group process and become aware of its application

– identify mental health concepts applicable in any nursing situations

– become familiar with adaptive coping mechanisms and maladaptive behaviors

– plan and implement nursing interventions to meet the psychosocial needs of clients

Acknowledgments

The support system formulated while in the process of writing always derives from many persons and sources. The assistance of each cannot always be identified but they have certainly played specific roles in helping the author toward completion of the manual.

I am grateful to our students with whom I have worked because without them the creation of this manual would never have given me the inspiration; to all nursing faculty members of Humber College of Applied Arts and Technology, Health Sciences Division, especially Joan Forsey, Zeny Manero, Sheila Money; to other colleagues from various learning institutions who in their desire to improve education have offered ideas in the testing and elaboration of the concepts.

Many thanks to Dean Jack Buckley, Associate Dean Marina Heidman, Director of Nursing, Anne Bender for their continued interest and support; and to Jocelyn Hezekiah, Director of Health Sciences, Grant McEwan College, for providing the initial intellectual inspiration of the first edition.

My appreciation to Sally Taylor for typing the manuscript and certainly to my friend, Barbara Riordan Massiah who provided the much needed emotional support during the moments of agony and ecstasy of writing.

1984   NdC

Student-Teacher Relationship

Norma S. de Castro, Ph.D.

As I view it, our relationship is one
That facilitates the personal and professional growth of one another.
If I am the teacher, I should know more than you
If you are the student, you are the recipient of this knowledge.
Perhaps this is the goal that is set for us,
Not by our choice but out of necessity.
However, you and I decided
To make this interaction a meaningful one;
An interaction that led to a relationship based on
  mutual respect for one another,
  reciprocal involvement,
  shared responsibility,
And together, we form an alliance.
With a deep sense of purpose and commitment
I am here because of you
To facilitate your potential growth to its maximum
That you may become the person you always wanted to be.
In your desire to learn, to know and understand,
You display eagerness, enthusiasm and delight,
Not to mention the apprehension and uncertainty
That you exhibit on numerous instances.
Like a newborn babe, you commit yourself to my care.
Like a nurturing significant mother, I hold you close to me.
Without me, this relationship cannot exist.
Without you, neither would it exist.
Together we come to a depth of knowing, accepting and caring.
Together we experience a timelessness in growth and need for each other.
Together we also risk losing sight of our educational goals.
Like any other relationship
Ours is not without any flaw.
We experience superficial togetherness;
We disagree and we argue;
We adhere to our own subjective values.
I rejected you and you rejected me
And we both risk losing one another.
But the humanness of our relationship
Led us to reassure one another.
We begin to appreciate how the other person feels and thinks.
Our time spent together in learning
Becomes indeed a memorable one,
And we can proudly say upon parting
That we were once a part of each other's lives.

CHAPTER 1

The Helping Relation

- Nurse-Client Interaction
- Nurse-Client Relationship
- Self Awareness
- Concept of Empathy

To sum up the qualities of a helping relation, it can be stated that human beings are deeply caring, understanding, accepting and available individual and can perceive the others as basically self-directing and responsible persons. Although he or she may not be always be this way as long as the person is open and comfortable in revealing his or her reactions to others, the person will continue to offer a helping relation. This is all to the good but the reality of life and emphasis of the qualities in itself may prompt the question of speaking only about the virtues of the helping relation and not the difficulties of it.

Carl Rogers discussed and expressed some of the difficulties of extending this caring to another as follows:

"Can I let myself experience positive attitudes toward the other person—attitudes of warmth, caring, liking, interest and respect? It is not easy. I find in myself and feel that I often see in others a certain amount of fear in these feelings. We are afraid that if we let ourselves freely experience these positive feelings toward another we may be trapped by them. They may lead to demand on us, or we may be disappointed in our trust, and these outcomes we fear. As a reaction we tend to build distance between ourselves and others—aloofness, a "professional attitude", an impersonal relationship. It is a real achievement when we can learn, even in a certain relationship or at a certain time in those relationships, that it is safe to care, that it is safe to relate to the other person for whom we have positive feelings."

The study of helping relation has become the core of most educational programs and the basic concepts of such relation are integrated throughout the curriculum. Although the growth in scientific research and understanding of human behaviors may have altered its principles, the application and the significance of the concept will continue to be the first requisite regardless of scientific advances, specifically in nurse-client relation which can be expressed in terms of related but distinguishable aspects of interaction, developmental phases, self-awareness and sympathy.

NURSE-CLIENT INTERACTION

Interaction is basic to all human relationships and it goes on constantly in human activity. Our present knowledge of human behavior, a term describing all human activity and responses, tells us that in order for man to survive, he must not only have various environments, but must maintain contact with these environments and through this total behavior, carry on an interaction with them which leads to some form of adaptation. Similarly related to this aspect is the nurse who is also in constant interaction with the environment attempting to meet his or her needs and adaptation, in addition to the peculiar interpersonal environment where the client and nurse must carry on an interchange with them. Thus, the process of interacting with the client becomes an integral part and characteristic pattern of nurse-client relationships. It is, therefore, helpful to note that both the client and the nurse feed into the whole interplay of forces which influence their behavioral responses in any given situation.

"Nurse-client interaction" then, refers to any nurse-client contact during which the nurse and the client have a reciprocal influence on each other, either verbally or non-verbally, positively or negatively, facilitating or inhibiting, but never neutral."

Significance of Interaction
- provide a maximum likelihood of success or failure in the care of the client
- aid or hinder the client in the process of adjustment as a result of illness status
- promote a sense of well being by maintaining self identity, dignity and sense of worth; or may promote dehumanization
- influence or deter the establishment of nurse-client relationship as the nurse and client move through the process of striving to know each other
- provide either positive or negative learning experience for both the client and the nurse

Tools of Interaction
- observation and communication skills
- self awareness
- nurse-client relation
- empathy

These will be further discussed.

PROCESS RECORDING

Definition:
"A Process Recording is a systematic method of collecting data prior to interpreting, analyzing, and synthesizing the data obtained."

Basic Premise:
1. All behavior has meaning
2. There is no such thing as non-behavior
3. All communication has meaning
4. There is no such thing as non-communication

Purpose:
1. To improve the quality of nursing care. This tool can be used objectively to review client communication, and the interaction between the nurse and the client, which results from each person's perception of the other.

   The nurse should be able to analyze the client's appearance, his or her motivation, the reason behind his or her behavior, and his or her communication, both overt and covert. From this analysis, the nurse should be able to plan further interactions and goals for same.

2. To develop the skill of the nurse to plan, structure and evaluate interpersonal relationships on a conscious level.

3. To lower the nurse's anxiety by improving his or her clinical practice, develop an awareness of verbal and non-verbal communication, thoughts and feelings in relationship to others and to focus attention and awareness on identifying nursing problems and problem solving.

EXPECTATION OF CONTENT IN PROCESS RECORDING INTERACTION STUDY

CLIENT: _____

TIME: _____

PLACE: _____

GOALS: _____

Nurse	Client	Comments and Evaluation

Column 1—The Nurse

1. State your communication skills

2. Thoughts and Feelings

   This column contains the thoughts and feelings you had *at the time of interaction*. It should *not* include those which are in retrospect or are a speculation.

   These will include, for example:

   a) re self   — *Feelings* like "felt own shoulders tensing up, made me feel uncomfortable."

                                  — *Thoughts* like "I'm scared."

   b) re client   — *Thoughts* like "I think this client is uncomfortable."

   c) re the environment   — *Thoughts* like "This room is dirty, is dark."

                                  — *Feelings* like "I want to leave this place now."

   There can be more than one thought or feeling at the time.

Column 2—The Client

1. State your client's responses, i.e. "I don't know, leave me alone."

2. State your client's behavior according to your perception, i.e. "client looking down, no eye contact, sad look on his/her face, appear apprehensive"

Column 3—Comments and Evaluation

1. State the type of communication techniques you utilized, i.e. giving recognition, validating, acceptance

2. State your interpretation of client's comments and behavior, i.e. "Mr. X was resentful of my talking to him; he became angry when I asked him further information; may be threatened by my questioning; stated "nobody cares for me anyway so why bother?""

Summary

1. Was the interaction therapeutic or non-therapeutic? In what way?

2. In retrospect, would you have handled the interaction similarly?

   If not, what would you have changed?

Exercise 1
INTERACTION PROCESS

Duration: 15 minutes

Direction: – Talk to a classmate or client for 5 minutes
            – Record your interaction according to the expected content of an interaction as previously stated in this section.
            – Then analyze the interaction.

Self	Other Person	Comments and Evaluation

Summary

_____

_____

_____

_____

4

NURSE-CLIENT RELATIONSHIP

The effectiveness of helping relation between the nurse and the client seem to be one of the recurrent concerns in the nursing profession as the changing role of the nurse is becoming increasingly complex. Yet one factor remains constant, the nurse-client relationship.

Nurse-client relationship may be described as a state of being mutually or reciprocally interested in each other, helping each other learn and grow through therapeutic interactions, structuring and guiding the relation toward common goals and in assisting the client meet his or her needs by use of knowledge and skills. It is a helping relation in which one person facilitates the personal development or growth of another to become a more mature, adaptive and integrated person.

It would seem, however, that while pursuing this changing role one might easily overlook some of the more basic ingredients of a relation that enhances its success and effectiveness and the ones that every client looks for—trust, feeling of being cared for, acceptance, recognition, respect, support and warmth.

To achieve this undertaking requires self-awareness, knowledge of human behavior, ability to communicate, establishment and maintenance of a therapeutic nurse-client relation. Though this may seem confusing and at first a hopeless task, willingness to learn without giving up in the face of failure will minimize the nurse's helplessness and he or she will begin to develop skills and function in the role of a therapeutic agent.

The phases of the nurse-client relation will provide convenient guides for assessment, planning, implementation and evaluation of the process of working closely with clients in any given setting. The nurse will attempt to recapture what occurred during the relationship, why it happened and how the client can be helped.

Phases of Nurse-Client Relationship

1. Orientation Phase

The orientation phase is the initial period in which the nurse and the client more or less get acquainted with each other. The client may not be too responsive to the nurse at this time and may test the nurse's concern and interest. The length of this phase and whether the interaction and the relationship will remain on this level will be influenced by several factors. The tasks of the orientation phase are:
- introduction of self, title, length of time to be spent with the client and clarification of roles and expectations
- creation of an environment which is conducive for interactions
- give information regarding the purpose and goals of interactions; time, place, length of interaction; and termination of nurse-client relationship
- orientation to routine and policies of the institution; explanation of treatment modalities, diagnostic tests
- give recognition to client as a person by addressing client with title such as Mr. or Mrs. and last name; allow client's preference in activities of daily living if possible
- initial assessment of client's needs and concerns
- exploration of own feelings

2. Working Phase

The working phase is the second stage of the nurse-client relationship which may be brief or extended, depending upon the hospital stay of the client, and it is a more structured period than the orientation phase. This stage is initiated with fairly well established rapport and some feeling of trust on the part of the client. The client may assume some initiative in interaction, awaits the nurse and manifests interest in the nurse. The client, however, may still test the nurse's limits of the relationship; become dependent upon the nurse; the client becomes more verbally expressive and is able to focus on concerns and problems; and the nurse usually serves as a sounding board for the client in clarifying thoughts and feelings.

During the phase, the following tasks can be pursued:
- gather more information for further assessment; clarification of previous information given
- assist in increasing the client's ability to verbalize; focus on problem areas
- assist client in exploring other ways of handling anxiety frustration, hostilities, and so forth
- promote client's self confidence by allowing independent functions; making some decisions; implementing and testing of planned actions; and evaluating the results of actions
- exploration of own reactions
- handle client's resistive behavior

3. Termination Phase

The termination phase is the last period of the nurse-client relationship which is evidenced by the client's working out own problems to the extent that the client no longer requires the intensive support of the nurse.

Termination phase is a gradual weaning process and if the relationship is to be resolved for any reason other than an indication by the client, anticipatory guidance is necessary. The conclusion of an ending relationship can be a complex process and usually engenders many mixed emotions, generally known as "anxiety separation". At times, the client may behave like he or she did during the orientation phase and/or may bring up new problems just as the nurse is concluding the relationship. The tasks to be accomplished in this phase are:
- summarization and evaluation of the nurse-client relationship
- confrontation of the reality of termination
- display more evidence of independent functions
- discussion of alternate ways of coping with the situation that caused the problem
- mutual exploration of thoughts and feelings about the termination phase

Exercise 2

THE NURSE'S ROLE IN MENTAL HEALTH

Duration: 10 minutes

Directions: Insert True or False before each of the following statements:

_____ 1. The nurse's role is to function in interpersonal relationships with individuals and with groups of clients.

_____ 2. The effectiveness of nursing care is not dependent upon the individual nurse's ability to interact.

_____ 3. The nurse as an observer should interview and interpret to the client.

_____ 4. The nurse as an observer cannot observe effectively as a participant.

_____ 5. It is not the duty of the nurse to intervene in interaction between two clients when they are arguing.

_____ 6. The nurse is not a strategic person who helps co-ordinate team relationships.

_____ 7. The nurse does clarify interrelationships of the various people in the ward society with the client.

_____ 8. The nurse as a leader should plan all activities for the client.

_____ 9. Conversation should be discouraged between clients at meal times.

_____ 10. The client should be fed as efficiently and quickly as possible.

_____ 11. Positive or learning situations cannot be gained at the meal table.

_____ 12. Many emotionally ill clients have utilized withdrawal because of their extreme sensitivity and anxiety in relation to other people.

_____ 13. The nurse as a counsellor should talk whenever the opportunity presents itself.

_____ 14. When the nurse does talk, it helps the client think through his/her problems and come to a decision which is helpful to him/her.

_____ 15. The nurse deals primarily with problems of physiological needs.

_____ 16. There is no need for the psychiatrist to work with the nurse.

_____ 17. It is the sole responsibility of the nurse to help the client deal in a more mature way as he or she relates with individuals and groups.

_____ 18. The nurse as a Patient Advocate does not look for or encourage her client to assume responsibility for his/her own care.

_____ 19. Clients should be allowed to set their own limits.

_____ 20. The nurse may be able to supply the client with a positive emotional experience which can substitute for one in which he or she has never before been able to share.

Exercise 3
NURSE-CLIENT RELATIONSHIP

1. Identify various nursing situations that may provide opportunities for interactions.

2. List the factors that may block or facilitate an interaction.

3. Identify and list some behavioral ploys that a client may utilize to test your interest and concerns.

4. Make a list of behaviors, including thoughts and feelings, that a client might have in reaction to the termination of a nurse-client relationship.

5. Cite an incident where you think you have experienced a meaningful nurse-client relation and state your reasons why you felt it was therapeutic or meaningful.

SELF-AWARENESS

Self-awareness is acknowledging the presence of thoughts and feelings and its corresponding behaviors. Looking at oneself in relation to the world, people think and act most of the time in terms of their own immediate feelings and inner world. Feelings as expressed through the unconscious, govern the individual far more than does the intellect. This is typical of the way feelings and thoughts operate in behavior, and man being creatures of habit and fearful of change, are constantly meeting resistance in attempts to control thoughts and how they feel.

In developing self-awareness this becomes an obstacle to bring the unconscious motivation to conscious level, thereby making the individual resistive. The process of self-awareness may be compared to a form of self-analysis. One must remember that one of the most difficult things in the world is to see oneself in a true and realistic perspective, to admit to oneself let alone to others, that one has faults.

Becoming aware of these set patterns and how it affects oneself and others, the individual can know more about his inner self and in doing so, he or she may facilitate or alter the self image that one holds on about oneself, thereby enriching his life and his relation to the environment. To develop some understanding and awareness of self requires conscious effort and patience, time and concentration to think and become aware over some of the behavior that one may consider virtues, how one perceives oneself, and the standards that have been imposed through past conditioning. Upon examination of one's behavioral patterns the individual may find that utilization of these habits may act as a defense for oneself.

Lack of developing self-awareness, gaining knowledge of what is happening inside the person, understanding one's own attitude, feelings, ideas that have been carried from within for many years can conceivably interfere with one's ability to evaluate other's feelings and to deal with them effectively. Anger, for example, toward someone may not be based on actions which might be mildly frustrating but rather upon previous experiences that happened and were not yet resolved in one's own thinking.

Such circumstances can be relieved by looking closely and carefully at situations which aroused such emotions and determine whether the reaction is just in terms of the situation or letting loose feelings from other situations. Such analysis can prevent unpleasant situations from occurring and will provide valuable information about the sources of our own feelings. The goal of self-awareness in normal interaction and relation is an attempt to understand our responses in terms of what they may mean to others who will have to deal with or interpret them. In other words, one should try to see oneself as others see them.

Self-understanding is a continuing process, requiring one to be aware of own needs and reactions in many great situations. There is some danger, of course, in the too analytical approach in which one may look for the hidden symbolic meaning in every feeling or reaction. One can easily become defensive and deny the existence of areas of difficulties and displace their feelings on others who are less able to defend themselves. There is little risk involved in developing insight and understanding as long as the goal is the sound healthy desire to improve one's relation with others. Similarly, no one can have full understanding of emotions of how they developed, of what purpose it serves and how it can be utilized to one's advantage.

Needless to say, man is not simply a collection of cultural and social roles, past experiences and biological influences. In addition, there is recognition of personality characteristics as distinct from others. The self has three major aspects, namely: how a person sees own self; how others see that person; and the actual self.

We would be limited in understanding ourself if it were not for the responses to us by other people and yet it is also difficult to know the impact of what our selves have on others and how they judge us. On measuring how a person sees himself, how he would like to be seen, and how others see him, studies revealed that most individuals see themselves somewhat more positively than others see them, while others tend to be more critical of themselves. Differences of opinions re: self by others, does not necessarily indicate that one is in serious error, but rather is due to limited exposure and sampling of one's own behavior.

Hence, self-awareness in the light of one's own past and present, can be more accurately sensitive than that of others and one can judge present behavior in terms of what has happened before, and he or she will be in a better position to evaluate one's ownself in terms of its growth.

Thus, self-awareness plays a major role in discussion of helping relation, communication and attitudes which greatly affect how others may respond to the individual.

THE SELF IMAGE

Duration: 10 minutes

Directions: Participants divide into a team of 2–4, sit in a circle and talk to each other by sharing some personal qualities with one another according to the following suggested dimensions:

- state physical attributes that you like best in yourself
- state personality traits that you like best in yourself
- state the skill or talent that you have and like

Complete this exercise and then turn to the next page.

1. How long did it take you to start sharing these qualities with the group? Why?

2. How many of you hesitated stating your positive qualities and instead gave the negative aspect of self? Why?

3. Did you find it difficult to share these qualities? If yes, why? If no, why not?

4. How do you feel now?

Exercise 5

ASSERTIVE SKILLS INVENTORY

Duration: 10 minutes

Direction: Please answer the following questions according to the way you normally would behave and communicate.

Put a check (✓) in one of the columns that best describes you. Honest answers are necessary.

	YES (usually)	NO (seldom)	SOMETIMES
1. Do you seek clarification when you are asked a question that is not clear?			✓
2. Do you ask a person to tell you how he/she feels about you?			✓
3. Is it difficult for you to talk to others?			✓
4. Do you find it hard to express your ideas when they differ from others?		✓	
5. Do you withhold topics that may hurt others?			✓
6. Do you have a tendency to dominate others in conversations?			✓
7. Do you confront others and discuss your feelings when they have hurt you?			✓
8. Do you fail to disagree due to fear of rejection?			✓
9. Do you fail to say "no" for fear of rejection?			✓
10. Do you become uncomfortable when someone compliments you?		✓	
11. Do you find it difficult to compliment others?		✓	
12. Is it difficult for you to trust others?			✓
13. Do you give others a chance to get to know you?			✓
14. While talking, are you aware how others are reacting to what you are saying?	✓		
15. Do you withdraw when someone upsets you?	✓		

CONCEPT OF EMPATHY

The other aspect of a relationship is the concept of empathy. It is not uncommon that when a client is distressed, nurses respond to this in terms of understanding the meaning of the turmoil at the moment and give reassurance. Although reassurance is a common and understandable response, it does not help the client to be told that the troubled feelings will do him or her any good, that one's worries have no basis in reality, or that other people have the same difficulties. Sympathetic reassurance may meet the need of the nurse to provide assistance, but one wonders if it ever offers more than temporary or superficial relief to the client who is being reassured. It is therefore important that nurses maintain a clear distinction between the meaning of sympathy and empathy. By definition, "empathy is the intellectual understanding of something in another person which is foreign to oneself" while "sympathy is the emotional understanding of another person's feelings".

The concepts of these two terms however, involves more than defining. "Empathy" implies that there is a close feeling with the client about his concerns; that one appreciates how the client inwardly feels and it does not mean that the client's thoughts, feelings and concerns becomes the nurse's problems. It excludes the process of identification where feelings and reactions which originated from the nurse's personal experiences and one that resemble the experiences of the client take over and to some extent becomes the object of responses without realizing it. The nurse as a human being will evoke some degree of involvement and will somehow display some emotional expression. Censoring the degree of emotional feeling and dealing with these feelings effectively and attempting to get to know the client and understand the nature of his or her concerns and illnesses, can serve a certain degree of empathy.

Simply stated, empathy implies that we "tune in" to the client's wave length and receive the message that the client is attempting to communicate without incorporating within us what the client has initiated; understanding the other from the other person's own frame of reference.

Attempting to experience the client's feelings intellectually and to remain objective is a difficult task and will require experience and a high level of accomplishment. By being too objective, one may under-react to the point of having no or limited feeling for and understanding of the client. Conversely, one may overly react and become too closely identified with the client and neither position will assist the client and may become detrimental instead.

Sympathy, on the other hand, being defined as an emotional understanding of another person's feeling, may limit or hinder the client's ability to express own's concerns and reinforce feelings of helplessness and worthlessness.

Both terms, however, suggest a caring attitude and reaching out to the other but sympathy denies the problem and to suppress it, while empathy will foster a process of working through an actual resolution of the problem by the client.

Empathy cannot be learned in theory only. It places high demands on self-awareness, objectivity, sensitivity, communication, respect and establishment of an emotional climate in which the client feels considered and respected. The tenets of empathy have to be practiced, have to be lived, and have to permeate the actual nurse-client relation in order to make the helping relation a meaningful one.

Suggested Readings

Burgess, A. W., *Psychiatric Nursing in the Hospital and the Community*. 3rd ed. Englewood Cliffs, Prentice-Hall Publishing Co., 1981

Carkhuff, R. et. al., *The Art of Helping III*. Amherst, Mass. Human Resource Development Press, 1977

Gerrard, B. et. al., *Interpersonal Skills for Health Professionals,* Reston, Virginia, Reston Publishing Co. Inc. A Prentice-Hall Co., 1980

Hays, J. S. and Larsen, K. H., *Interacting with Patients*. New York, MacMillan Co., 1969

Kreig, H. and Perko, J., *Psychiatric and Mental Health Nursing: Commitment to Care and Concern*. 2nd ed. Reston, Virginia, Reston Publishing Co., A Prentice-Hall Co., 1983

Kyes, J. and Hofling, C. K., *Basic Psychiatric Nursing Concepts,* 4th ed., Philadelphia/Toronto, J. B. Lippincott Co., 1980

Stuart, G. W. and Sundeen, S. J., *Principles and Practice of Psychiatric Nursing*. 2nd ed. St. Louis/Toronto. The C. V. Mosby Co., 1983

Exercise 6
EMPATHY

Duration: 10 minutes

Direction: Identify the statements that reflect the concept of emphatic responding.

1. I know what you mean. I felt that way too.

2. You are feeling anxious because you are worried about your condition.

3. You will feel better soon.

4. You feel alone and you miss your family.

5. That is an awful feeling. I don't blame you for feeling that way.

6. I will stay with you for a while.

7. It is not that bad. Your family will be here soon.

8. I am not sure that I understand what you are saying.

9. It is terrible to feel powerless.

10. You feel powerless because you do not have control over your situation.

CHAPTER 2

Communication

- Modes of Communication
- Variables Affecting Communication Process
- Communication Techniques

"I know you believe that you understand what you think I said, but I am not sure that you realize that what you heard is not what I meant."

Communication is a broad term that can be defined in many different ways as it means every kind of behavior in all areas of human life. It has various meanings and interpretations to different people and depending on how it is used.

Hence, it is not uncommon that the reader will come across varied definitions of communication and it is beyond the scope of this workbook to outline such variations. Instead, only the most simplified version of communication will be presented here, but enough to give you the flavor of current thinking in this field.

Simply stated, communication implies that message is understood by both sender and receiver. Given the reality of differences in life experiences, this is impossible, as communication is an ongoing, dynamic, complex process. It is not merely an act of sending messages from one person to another but the messages must be mutually understandable to both sender and receiver; it must have the same meaning to both and feedback should be received in order to complete the process of communication.

MODES OF COMMUNICATION

1. *Communication as Behavior*

    It has been shown that since the beginning of time organisms, man or animal has acquired and developed signals as modes of communicating to each other. In this context, communication consists of signals made by one organism that have meaning for other organisms and thus affect their behavior. Although language using words is the richest form of communication, much of our communication does not hang on the meaning of words. Instead, we communicate our thoughts and feelings. The way we look at other people, how we stare at them, how we nod our heads, the gestures with which we punctuate our actions or speech, the way we sit and even our style of talking and walking, all communicate something to other people. This is also referred to as non-verbal communication, and currently known as kinesic communication.

2. *Communication as a System of Operation*

    It is a process whereby a step by step logical progression of messages must be established in order to make ideas clear and exchange of information to occur. It involves "encoding" which is the process of translating ideas into an appropriate message to the receiver; and "decoding", the process of translating the message of the sender by the receiver to determine its meaning. The messages of both the sender and receiver can be verbal or non-verbal.

3. *Communication as an Interaction*

It is a dynamic reciprocal process that takes into account the experiences and feelings of both the sender and receiver. Meaning of communication does not occur simply because words are spoken. Both the sender and the receiver attempt to know each other's psychological frame of reference; when, how, and under what circumstances one is required or expected to behave or communicate. This flexibility allows both individuals to move from one level of communication to another.

4. *Communication as a Social Process*

Unlike the animals, man has developed a way of communicating with each other through the use of language in which spoken and written words are used to convey meaning. The formation of the individual's personality, character structure, perception of self and the world, his or her role in it, is in part, developed as a result of social communication during the growth and development process.

Language and communication although related do not mean the same thing. Language differs from culture to culture, from age groups to other groups, social class, occupation or profession, which may have their own vocabulary. The language used by these groups or cultures provides members with a commonly accepted way of describing their experiences and communicating them to others.

5. *Communication as a Listening Activity*

Courses in communication still tend to emphasize on how to speak and write effectively rather than on the effective reception and assimilation of ideas. People confuse hearing with listening believing that because hearing is a natural function, then listening must be effortless. On the contrary, listening is hard work, requires increased psychological functions, conscious effort to penetrate the physical and psychological distractions and makes the unconscious activity of hearing into a conscious act of listening. Human nature makes us want to hear only what pleases us and to reject that which does not. Therefore, we are prone to listen only to ideas which are in accord with our own viewpoint and to discount those we find disagreeable. To listen effectively is one form of communication where one needs to guard against the tendency of emotional censorship and clearly receive the emotional message that one is conveying. Non-verbal language is often missed or misinterpreted because of ineffective listening skills. People give out non-verbal signs as they talk; gestures, pauses, hesitations may tell more about the real message than the verbal responses, and visual observation of body language reflects how one feels about what is being said and not just what one thinks. All it takes basically is an awareness that listening is a difficult demanding function which demands care and effort, both when one listens and when one talks.

LISTEN

When I ask you to listen to me
  and you start giving advice
  you have not done what I asked.

When I ask you to listen to me
  and you begin to tell me why I shouldn't feel that way,
  you are trampling on my feelings.

When I ask you to listen to me
  and you feel you have to do something to solve my problem,
  and you have failed me, strange as that may seem.

Listen! All I asked, was that you listen.
  not talk or do—just hear me.
Advice is cheap: 10 cents will get you both Dear Abby and
  Billy Graham in the same newspaper.
And I can do for myself; I'm not helpless.
  Maybe discouraged and faltering, but not helpless.

When you do something for me that I can and need to do
  for myself, you contribute to my fear and weakness.

But, when you accept as a simple fact that I do feel what I feel,
  no matter how irrational, then I can quit trying to convince
  you and can get about the business of understanding what's
  behind this irrational feeling.
And when that's clear, the answers are obvious and I
  don't need advice.
Irrational feelings make sense when we understand what's
  behind them.

Perhaps that's why prayer works, sometimes, for some people
  because God is mute, and he doesn't give advice or
  try to fix things. "They" just listen and let you
  work it out for yourself.

So, please listen and just hear me. And if you want to
  talk, wait a minute for your turn; and I'll listen to you.

                                                    Anonymous

VARIABLES AFFECTING COMMUNICATION PROCESS

1. Intrapersonal framework of each participant—involves perception of self and others; how one feels about oneself; feeling and thinking state at the time; what occurs prior to an interaction or communication will affect one's feelings and readiness of the receiver to understand the message; past experiences of the participants.
2. Context in which communication occurs—includes the physical and psychological environment— for example: time, place, setting, climate, appropriateness of communication; readiness of the receiver; what the receiver is doing, feeling and thinking at the time.
3. Encoding and decoding a message—explores the intent of the message; how the message is transmitted; how the message is received; and the feedback mechanism.
4. Speed and Pacing—is related to the amount of information to be given at one time; channels of communication—for example: verbal or written communication; information-processing capacities of the listener; receiver's rate of comprehension.
5. Communication skills—involves clarity of the message, either through verbal or written; is the language understandable; appropriate use of words; focus on communication or interaction.
6. Acknowledgement of different meanings—recognizing that verbal and non-verbal language have different meaning to different people—for example: culture, roles of the sender and the receiver, status, various age groups; manner of speaking and tone of voice and gestures.

Barriers to Effective Communication

Verbal	Non-verbal
talking too fast	attitudes
poor choice of words	prejudice
improper sentence structure	preoccupation
differences in language level	negative feelings
disorganized thoughts	selective listening
failure to respond	defensive listening
failure to understand	gestures that convey lack of interest
absence of feedback	overidentification
failure to focus	projection
inaccurate interpretation	reaction to appearance
inaudible voice perception	inappropriate facial expression
external stimuli	judgemental conclusion
need to talk	
generalization	

Factors that Facilitate Effective Communication

listening

empathy

consistency

gestures that convey interest and concern

non-judgemental attitude

clarity of message

all expression at client's own pace

establish climate conducive to communication

focus on client rather than own experience

accurate perception

use of communication techniques

COMMUNICATION TECHNIQUES

The word "therapeutic" means to heal or cure and communication techniques are methods or tools used to accomplish the specific as well as the overall goals of nursing interventions. It differs from social interaction or social communication in that therapeutic communication consists of specific sequential acts of communicating for the purpose of maintaining, promoting and restoring health. The techniques of communications are goal directed and are used to guide the development of a reciprocal and meaningful dialogue and to assist the nurse to achieve the goal of one to one relationship.

The thrust of therapeutic communication techniques is directed toward the "here and now" problems of the client. Nurses quite often engage in small social talk rather than get involved in the client's problems. These habitual modes of communicating with others can only evoke an automatic stereotype response which is devoid of meaning. To be therapeutic, the nurse should not remain in this level of communication and needs to break through the client's barrier to self disclosure. It is not uncommon that at the beginning of an interaction, both the nurse and the client may feel comfortable in utilizing stocks of small talk as a prelude to a more meaningful communication.

Communication techniques are means to an end and not ends within themselves. Not all nurses will feel comfortable using these techniques and will need assistance and practice in developing these skills. At times, it is well not to consider using these communication techniques if it is going to block the interaction process. For example, rigid and excessive inappropriate use of "reflective technique" on a client who is seeking answers to a simple question will evoke frustration and hostility. One of many common comments by clients subjected to the reflective or non-directive techniques is that they never get a straightforward answer or that their questions are often answered with a question. Nurses are encouraged to develop and use any of the techniques that they feel comfortable with, with much discretion and judgment. Adeptness in the use of therapeutic communication techniques, however, does not necessarily guarantee success of the expected outcome without obvious evidence of caring attitude, that is, the ability to care for and about the other.

In the section which follows, communication techniques considered therapeutic and non-therapeutic are given with examples and these techniques are also tools of the interviewing process.

Communication Techniques

Therapeutic Techniques	Examples
Use silence	– (sitting quietly and appearing interested but no verbal communication)
Give recognition	– Good evening John, or Mr. . . . . . – Thank you for helping around . . . – You look relaxed this evening
Demonstrate acceptance	– Yes . . . – Uh hmm. . . . . . – I follow what you are saying
Offer self	– I will spend some time with you – I will go out for a walk with you – How can I help you?

Therapeutic Techniques	*Examples*
Give broad openings	– What would you like to talk about?
	– Where would you like to begin?
	– How do you feel now?
Offer general leads	– What happened?
	– And then . . . . .
	– Go on . . . .
Place event in time and sequence	– When did you start feeling this way?
	– Was this before or after . . . . ?
	– What were your thoughts before this?
Make observations	– You appear angry
	– You look uncomfortable when . . .
	– I notice you are clenching your fists
Encourage description of observation	– How does it feel to be anxious?
	– What is the voice telling you?
	– Have you had similar experiences like this before?
Restate	Client: I stayed awake all night
	Nurse: You have difficulty sleeping
	Client: I don't know whether I should go out with the group as I don't have any clothes and my mother might visit me.
	Nurse: You really do not wish to go if you are not properly dressed
	You wish to join the group if you are sure your mother is not coming to visit you
Reflection	Client: Do you think I should go?
	Nurse: Do you think you should?
	Client: My mother might be disappointed
	Nurse: And this makes you feel angry?
Focus on statement	– Let us talk more about this incident
	Client: Last night I really enjoyed the party
	Nurse: You said your mother might be disappointed
Explore	– Tell me more about that
	– What does your mother do when she gets disappointed?
	– How do you react to her then?

Communication Techniques—*Continued*

Therapeutic Techniques	*Examples*
Seek clarification	– I do not follow what you are saying
	– What are you trying to tell me?
	– How do you behave when you get angry?
Present reality	– I hear no voices
	– That was the radio
	– Your mother is not here. You are in the hospital
Give information	– You are in the hospital
	– Your mother will come during visiting hours which are from . . . . . to . . . . .
	– This medication will help you settle your nerves
Voice doubt	– I find that hard to believe
	– Do you really think she will be disappointed or will be glad?
	– Isn't that unusual?
Seek consensual validation	– Are you telling me that your mother gets angry when she comes and you are not around?
	– And as a result you get very hostile?
Verbalize the implied	Client: I cannot talk to you or anyone. You are all the same.
	Nurse: Is it your feeling that no one understands you?
	Client: My mother and my girl friend always tell me what to do
	Nurse: Is it your feeling that women are controlling?
Attempt to translate into feelings	Client: It's hopeless and I will not bother you anymore
	Nurse: Are you suggesting that you feel useless and desire to give up?
	– That must be frustrating
Suggest collaboration	– Maybe you and I can discuss further what makes you feel this way
Summarize interaction	– You said that . . . .
	– We have discussed . . . .
Formulate plan of action	– What can you do to express your anger constructively?
	– When this happens again, how would you handle it?

Communication Techniques—*Continued*

Non-Therapeutic Techniques	*Examples*
Giving reassurance	– Everything will be alright – Don't worry about that – You did all that you could
Giving approval	– I am glad that you . . . . – That is really good – You did quite well
Rejecting	– I do not wish to discuss this any further – Let us talk of something else
Disapproving	– I wish you did not . . . . . . – How many times did I tell you not to . . . .
Agreeing	– I agree that . . . . – You did it
Giving advice	– Maybe you should . . . . . . – This is the best way to . . . . .
Probing	– Now tell me about . . . . . – How is your sex life?
Challenging	– How can you be the Prime Minister? – If you are depressed, how can you function?
Testing	– Do you know what place this is? – Do you still feel that you are the Prime Minister? – Where are you now?
Making stereotyped comments	– Things will be better – It's really nice outside – How are you? You are looking great
Giving literal responses	Client: I am a disciple sent by God Nurse: St. Peter or St. Paul? Client: I am here to spread the Gospel Nurse: Gather the other clients then for group therapy and you can spread your gospel
Requesting an explanation	– Why do you think that you are a disciple? – Why do you feel that way? – Why did you do that?
Belittling expressed feelings	– I know what you mean. I feel that way sometimes – Everybody feels depressed every now and then

24

Communication Techniques—*Continued*

Non-Therapeutic Techniques	*Examples*
Interpreting	– What you are saying is . . . .
	– Perhaps unconsciously you want to . . . . . .
Introducing unrelated topic	Client: I wonder if my husband will be here before surgery
	Nurse: Did you go away for the summer?
Using denial	Client: Perhaps I have cancer
	Nurse: Don't be silly. Not all surgery is for cancer

Suggested Readings

Blondis, M. N. and Jackson, B., *Non-Verbal Communication with Patients*. New York. A Wiley Medical Publication, 1977

Collins, Mattie, *Communication in Health Care,* 2nd ed., St. Louis. The C. V. Mosby Co., 1983

Edwards, B. J. and Brilhart, J. K., *Communication in Nursing Practice,* St. Louis. The C. V. Mosby Co., 1981

Gerard, B. et. al., *Interpersonal Skills for Health Professionals,* Reston, Virginia. Reston Publishing Co., A Prentice Hall Co, 1980

Hays, J. S. and Larsen, K. H., *Interacting with Patients,* New York. MacMillan Co., 1969

Kreigh, H. and Perko, J., *Psychiatric and Mental Health Nursing: Commitment to Care and Concern.* 2nd ed. Reston, Virginia. Reston, Publishing Co., A Prentice Hall Co., 1983

Wilson, H. and Kneisl, C., *Psychiatric Nursing.* 2nd ed., Menlo Park, California. Addison Wesley Publishing Co., 1983

Exercise 7

NON-VERBAL COMMUNICATION

Duration: 15 minutes

Direction: Turn to the person next to you and talk to each other for 3–5 minutes. The subject matter is unimportant. After the stated length of time, stop and tell your partner what you have noticed about the other's non-verbal behavior. List the non-verbal behavior that you have observed, both you and your partner.

SELF   **PARTNER**

1. _____   _____

2. _____   _____

3. _____   _____

4. _____   _____

5. _____   _____

Interpret the possible reasons for these non-verbal behaviors.

_____

_____

_____

_____

_____

_____

_____

Exercise 8

THE ACT OF LISTENING

Duration: 20 minutes

Direction: Form a small circle with 8–10 participants. State your name or give a fictitious name (if the participants are familiar to you) and say something about yourself. Then the next person on your left repeats your name and what you said about yourself. Continue repeating the exercise from the left until each participant has stated all that has been said so far and finally the last participant adds his or her own name.

Complete this exercise then proceed to the next page.

– How much of what was said did you remember?

– What non-verbal behaviors have you observed?

– Who among the participants left an impression on you? Why?

– At what point of the exercise did you quit listening? Why?

Exercise 9

OBSERVATION

Duration: 10 minutes

Direction: Insert True or False before each of the following statements.

_____ 1. Change in behavior is one of the most striking indications of adaptive and maladaptive responses.

_____ 2. It is important for those who nurse the emotionally ill to ignore symptoms of behavior.

_____ 3. Having a better understanding of the significance of the nurse's observations, the doctor can make a more accurate diagnosis and a better plan of treatment.

_____ 4. In emotionally ill patients, the most easily observed symptoms relate to behavior.

_____ 5. Symptoms are easy to observe because they are only objective in origin.

_____ 6. Accurate observation and recording are simple and easy.

_____ 7. An understanding of client's behavior requires recognition of subjective aspects.

_____ 8. The nurse should hurry through the admission procedure to get the client settled as soon as possible.

_____ 9. Bruises and lacerations noted during the admission bath should be charted only if they are of a serious nature.

_____ 10. Not every contact with a client is an opportunity to observe.

_____ 11. As a participant observer, the nurse scrutinizes only the client's behavior, not her own.

_____ 12. The personality of the nurse affects her observations.

_____ 13. Observations can be influenced by the relationship between the nurse and the client's doctor.

_____ 14. Clients feel uncomfortable if a nurse obviously sits and watches them.

_____ 15. Recreational activity with the client as well as having therapeutic value for the client enables the nurse to observe his/her reactions.

Exercise 10

COMMUNICATION TECHNIQUES—I

Duration: 15 minutes

Direction: Please match Column A with Column B

Column A
Statements

_____ Good morning, Mr. Smith. I notice that you've combed your hair.

_____ I'll stay here with you.

_____ Where would you like to begin?

_____ Tell me about it.

_____ What seemed to lead up to . . . ?

_____ You appear tense.

_____ What happens when you feel anxious?

Patient: I can't sleep. I stay awake all night.

_____ Nurse: You have difficulty sleeping.

Patient: Do you think I should tell the doctor?

_____ Nurse: Do *you* think you should?

_____ This point seems worth looking at more closely.

_____ Tell me more about that.

_____ My purpose in being here is . . . .

_____ I'm not sure that I follow you.

_____ I see no one else in the room

_____ Really?

_____ What are your feelings in regard to . . . ?

Patient: I'm empty.

_____ Nurse: Are you suggesting that life seems without meaning?

_____ Perhaps you and I can discuss it and discover what produces your anxiety

_____ During the past hour you and I have discussed . . . . .

_____ What could you do to let your anger out harmlessly?

_____ I wouldn't worry about . . . .

_____ I'm glad that you . . . .

_____ I don't want to hear about . . . .

_____ I'd rather you wouldn't . . . .

_____ Just listen to your doctor and take part in activities. You'll be home in no time.

Patient: I have nothing to live for.

_____ Nurse: Everybody gets down in the dumps

Column B
Communication Techniques

1. Restating
2. Reflecting
3. Focusing
4. Exploring
5. Giving information
6. Seeking clarification
7. Presenting reality
8. Voicing doubt
9. Accepting
10. Offering self
11. Giving broad openings
12. Offering general leads
13. Placing the event in time or sequence
14. Making observations
15. Encouraging description of perception
16. Encouraging evaluation
17. Attempting to translate into feelings
18. Suggesting collaboration
19. Summarizing
20. Encouraging formulation of a plan of action
21. Making stereotyped comments
22. Reassuring
23. Giving approval
24. Rejecting
25. Disapproving
26. Belittling feelings expressed

Exercise 11

COMMUNICATION TECHNIQUES—II

Duration: 10 minutes

Direction: Identify the most appropriate specific communication techniques (lettered items) to the type of response a nurse might make to a client (numbered items).

Column I

_____ 1. You're coming along fine.

_____ 2. Perhaps you and I can discuss what produces your anxiety.

_____ 3. Where would you like to begin?

_____ 4. What does the voice seem to be saying?

_____ 5. Isn't that unusual?

_____ 6. This situation seems worth looking at more closely.

_____ 7. Tell me more about it.

_____ 8. I follow what you said.

_____ 9. Do you think you will feel better if you go home?

_____ 10. How would you take care of your family?

Column II

A. Posing a related problem

B. Posing a related question

C. Voicing doubt

D. Offering general leads

E. Reassuring

F. Suggesting collaboration

G. Encouraging description of perception

H. Accepting

I. Give broad opening

J. Focusing

CHAPTER 3

Group Process

- Group Structure
- Group Operation
- Membership Role
- Leadership Style
- Group Dynamics
- Group Experiences in Psychiatry and Mental Health Settings

The influence of man's social interaction in shaping his behavior and his contribution in social relation constitute a system of patterned relation which is the human group itself. The interaction duly recognizes that man is typically goal-directed from birth on and is uniquely endowed with capacity to learn human relation in group and learn to accept consequences of human actions in determining behavior.

The influence of people on one another is a group process, while universal in commonality, there are differences as well. Consequently, we become more aware of the impact of the group in forming interpersonal relations, setting of personal goals, in bringing about intended changes in behavior, work performance and problem solving skills.

Group has been defined by leading authorities as collection of individuals in which the relationship is necessary to the satisfaction of their individual needs; a collection of individuals working toward a common goal through cooperation.

Groups may begin in many ways. It can be formed spontaneously or as a result of a planned pattern of action, but regardless of the factors underlying the formation of a group, there are certain features essential to the existence of a group—common goal, membership, communication network, social climate, group standard and organizational structure.

GROUP STRUCTURE

1. *Common Goal*

The identification of the need or problem is the first step in the structure or formation of a group. An objective or goal within a group is a vital concern to members, organizers and for the purpose of evaluating the results of the groups' efforts. The goal may vary from that of an exchange of ideas to a specific plan of action but the group will not begin to function effectively without a clear understanding of the goal or its purpose. The determination of purpose will assist members to understand their own roles and their own attitude toward the problem to be solved or needs to be met. The formulation of a group goal requires that personal goals held by individual members be somewhat transformed into a single goal for the group and that this goal be capable of steering group activities. The emphasis on group goal is not intended to exclude the importance of the individual's personal goal and welfare but merely a caution to keep group goal in focus and within the boundary of achievement. When the wide variety of social and personal goals and needs that may be presented are considered, the work or task of the group will be accomplished. It is of great significance then that the goal of the group is clear, understandable, important and achievable.

2. Membership Participation

It is apparent that each person is a member of a seemingly endless number of groups, beginning from groups formed by family, friends, schools, organizations to which the person belongs and other affiliations that he or she have.

Interactions, the essential element in group behavior, may be minimal or maximal, depending on how much the person's energies are vested, their feelings about the group, whether they feel accepted or rejected, and how much freedom they have in interaction. Each member has needs and forces motivating and driving him or her towards group involvement. Hence the motivations, needs and experiences of members are constant influences in group process and the individual's own needs can dominate the group activities if the conditions are right and the pressures strong.

The strength of the pressure which can be exerted by a group is the result of its organizational strength and the attractiveness of the group to its members.

An understanding of the psycho-social nature of the group in relation to the needs and personal goals which are operative within each member is necessary to prevent digression and facilitate group function.

3. Communication Network

The important consideration would seem to be whether members can communicate and cooperate effectively in setting goals and sharing common interest in the accomplishment of group tasks while meeting the needs of each group member. It is well known that many factors contribute to the communication patterns and among them are the obvious factors of common language, thought processes, channels of communication, organizational structure, emotional climate, interpersonal feelings and attitudes, and even variables arising out of the personalities of the group members. Members and leaders need to listen, to understand and to accept expression of facts, needs and ideas to establish effective communication and meaningful interaction.

Other factors that require consideration which affect members' interrelationships are the elements of authority, status, power, physical arrangements, atmosphere of cooperation and competition. If communication network is not clearly defined and is not generally consistent with the personal reactions of group members, communication patterns become an impediment to effective group process.

4. Social Climate

Any group which attempts to obtain cooperation and involvement of group members need to be concerned about the social climate of the group. Group members who are threatened, frustrated, and feel the need to defend themselves will be more engrossed with that problem than with the stated group tasks or goals. The social climate therefore is the determiner of the communication level that exists among the members and the success of the group work.

An atmosphere of acceptance, permissiveness and social interaction are of basic importance for all aspects of group process. By acceptance is meant that each individual be accorded respect and status of belonging to a cohesive group, and permissiveness means freedom to express any ideas and feelings for consideration by the group with awareness that all members will attempt to understand and continue to accept each other in spite of their differences. The extent to which the social climate of the group will be created will also be largely dependent on the leader. As well, differences in social climate exist and it also varies according to the type of leadership provided.

5. Group Standard

The simple explanation of the process involved in this task is to lay out the steps which will be followed to achieve the stated group goals or tasks. Group standard or norms involves setting of rules, code of ethics, topics to be discussed, procedures to be utilized, length of time and mode of self expressions.

6. *Organizational Structure*

The organizational structure are concepts which define the nature of the group and assist a group toward its goal. Groups may be formal or informal, official or unofficial, approved or disapproved, organized or disorganized, task-centered or growth centered. Each of these facts about a group can change its functions, objectives and methods of operations. Hence, the organizational structure differs from group to group and is dependent on the type of group in existence, its goals, diversity of membership and social mobility.

GROUP OPERATION

1. *Group Formation Phase*

This is the initial and early stage of group formation. It involves orientation to the structural organization of the group, introduction of group members, development of objectives and/or clarification of the stated purpose or objectives of the group. The group will not be able to develop smoothly and function effectively without a clear understanding of the group goals, purposes or objectives. Hence, confusion, conflicts and difficulties of its purpose can usually be traced back to the formation process of the group.

This stage also provides opportunity to determine group members' level of aspiration and assist members to understand their roles in relation to the goal to be achieved and in setting group standards.

Other significant variables such as age, gender, needs and problems of the group members, frequence and length of group work requires special consideration during this stage of formation based on the purpose of the group.

2. *Group Interaction Phase*

At the initial stage of group interaction, members may covertly and overtly express frustrations, conflicts, thoughts and feelings. Members are cautiously courteous to each other, inhibited in self expression, may distrust other members and project their own feelings to others, may appear uninvolved and resistive to the goals stated. Although this phase attempts to facilitate feeling of permissiveness, the exchange of ideas and sharing of experiences among the entire group, group effort and decision making, the progression of group process is not an easy task due to members' attitude, expression of feelings, opinions, testing of ideas and behaviors.

Group interaction occurs at all phases and at all times, and it may be viewed as the background of the total process in the operation of groups. The nature and intensity of group interactions, however, take varying fashion depending on the social climate, interaction pattern already in existence, cohesiveness and purpose of the group. For example, in a group therapy process where group cohesiveness has been established, expression of hostilities are encouraged and inappropriate behaviors are discouraged, and both are dealt with directly by the group. In other group situations, group interaction may be focused in mobilizing energy for accomplishing the group goals.

3. *Group Cohesion Phase*

Cohesiveness may be further described as the "morale, the togetherness of a group" and "the sharing of understanding of purpose and function of a group".

At this point, the stage of cohesion may require some length of time for group members to become acquainted and display accepting attitudes of one member to another.

As members work together in establishing rapport, they begin to interact more freely, develop some fondness and affection for one another, become more friendly, display mutual respect and understanding and concern for one another, begin to express self more freely and continue to function together in the accomplishment of the objectives.

Many authorities in group process have equated the degree of group productivity to cohesiveness of the group. Many people perceive cohesiveness to be a measure of the success of the organizational structure of a group. Cohesive groups, groups with high morale, may be able to withstand greater pressure, deprivation and difficult situations than groups with low morale but is not necessarily the most effective group in accomplishing its tasks. The state of cohesiveness can affect many other factors vital to the ultimate success of the group. As previously stated, cohesiveness has its positive and negative component, is descriptive of group climate and attitudes but is not predictive of the effectiveness of the group. Such situations may be useful to the group leader in selected situations or in areas such as psychiatry to ensure fulfillment of therapeutic goals; or in any other group where a divisive force, the negative component of cohesiveness, is quite obvious that lead to non-productivity.

4. *Group Dissolution Phase*

This phase begins as the objectives or purposes of the group are near completion, and inevitably the termination of the existing group relationship. The achievement of the group tasks produce both positive and negative feelings for members. Positive attitude about self and the tasks are developed and concomittant with these feelings are the experienced feelings of loss. The type of termination and how it will be handled by the group will depend upon the objectives, the intensity of the experience, cohesiveness and the type of participants. In task-oriented groups, termination may occur with minimal emotional reactions. For others, depending upon the nature of the group involved in the process, the discomfort level of loss and anxiety generated by the separation becomes extremely high. For example, the establishment of plan for termination of a group process in group therapy sessions, is more difficult to achieve than in a one-to-one individual counselling.

MEMBERSHIP ROLE

"Role" may be described as a set of behaviors expected of a person who occupies a given status; and "status" is a position or function occupied by a person. According to social psychologists, status is a motivating force in all areas of life. It is an advanced type of esteem which refers to prestige, specific rights, privileges, duties reserved for members or persons with groups, organizations and the like. Groups generally recognize selected and specific roles, for example, chairperson, recorder, observer, specialist, and identify individual members to fill these roles. Membership roles may have official or unofficial status within the group but nevertheless, all group members, members with selected key roles as well as the leader are all responsible in fulfilling their role function in relation to goal achievement and group maintenance functions.

Benne and Sheates identified and clarified effective group behavior and group functions which contribute to productivity and morale in groups and the accomplishment of its goals. In their classification, all group members assumes the identified behaviors and functions in varying proportion.

1. Group Tasks Roles—are those which help the group accomplish its work or goals and is related to the socio dimension of the group. The initiation of action, development and evaluation of plans and its implementation are the task centered responsibilities. Examples of the tasks roles or functions are:
   - *initiating:* suggesting new ideas or activities to mobilize group work; proposing new solutions; suggesting new strategies in defining problem or organization of plan
   - *regulating:* defining progress of discussion; re-stating goals; raising questions about direction of discussion; probing for meaning of statements and discussions; summarizing and setting time for discussion; focusing and guiding discussion; orientating new members about discussion
   - *informing and clarifying:* providing relevant facts and information; relating pertinent personal information; elaborating on comments; asking for relevant facts and information; seeking expression of opinions; clarifying of suggestions and ideas
   - *supporting:* creating emotional climate to promote harmony; relieving tension and facilitating group work
   - *evaluating:* assisting group to evaluate decision, goals, procedures, progress; feasibility of application of new ideas or suggestions; summarizing group consensus; coordinating relatedness of ideas and suggestions; interpreting and drawing together group conclusions

2. Group Building and Maintenance Roles—are those which assist to build relationship and cohesiveness in the group to complete the group tasks and is related to the psychic dimension of the group. Examples of these roles are:
   - *encouraging:* warmth, friendliness, giving praise and support to other members; displaying acceptance of others' ideas and behavior; asking others' opinion
   - *mediating:* promoting harmony; compromising; concilliating during disputes
   - *expediting:* gate-keeping; providing opportunities for members to contribute; avoiding and preventing dominance of discussion; suggesting time limit for discussion of certain topics
   - *listening:* attempting to understand others' point of view; accepting ideas of others; a listener; displaying group solidarity
   - *relieving tension:* assisting others and rewarding when members express opinons; diverting attention during tense moments; facilitating expression of strong feelings
   - *standard setting:* focusing on group procedures, rules and ethics; assisting to select topics for discussion

LEADERSHIP STYLE

Leadership role is the designated central figure within the structure of the group. There is no single method of selecting and appointing of leader for a group which will guarantee effective functioning of the group. Although there is no universal set of functions attributed to the responsibility of the leader, most research and theory have concluded that the environment, purpose, needs and structure of the group at a particular time are the determining factors in the functions of the leader and these undoubtedly also provide for the role differentiation or styles of leadership.

Various types of leadership have been examined with varied concepts of what the leader is and what he or she does in group situations. Inherent in all studies and discussion of leadership is the notion that there are responsibilities and functions which must be performed by all leaders. That is:

- initiate actions that help the group achieve its purpose

- assist and define membership roles

- establish group goals; provide information

- clarify group interactions; attend to human relation concerns

- maintain the group as an entity to solve or complete tasks

- interpret and draw conclusions

- evaluate group performance

While the above are the basic functions and tasks of the leader, they are also issues for each group member.

The leader is a member of the group although he or she is often looked upon as the most important factor in the operation of the group. Leadership may be assumed by the person himself or herself, may be appointed and or selected by group members. The group members are the other side of the coin of leadership and both are responsible for goal achievement and group maintenance, and its success depends upon the joint efforts of both. A leader in one group may be follower in other groups; conversely, a member in one group may become a leader in another.

The concept of leadership styles is deeply rooted in the work of Lewin and the widely known classical types are: a) authoritarian b) democratic c) laissez-faire. These types of leadership have been modified by most research authorities since the original formulation by Lewin. Frequently, there is overlapping of the characteristics and each type may contain some elements of each category. The following table provides an outlined characteristic of the classical types of leadership.

	Authoritarian	Democratic	Laissez-faire
Group Goal	- uses personal power to determine goals, objectives and actions - assign tasks to group members	- facilitate group participation - responsibility and authority are shared with members	- allows group to develop as members desire - deliberate lack of direction or control over goals
Social Climate	- dictatorial concept - little recognition of member as person - does not act with consent and approval from member - members in constant conflict with one another - coercive methods dominate - limited freedom of self expression from members - tense and controlled atmosphere	- group centered person - facilitate process; freedom to change; members are helped to become full functioning - personal satisfaction and provides reward - development by self interest - leaders usually chosen by group - power is derived from group - relaxed and informal atmosphere	- boredom, frustration - aggressive, hostile - climate may be imposed by members for development of group - power and authority are loose - permissive atmosphere - members assume responsibilities
Personality	- insist on rules and conformity - does not seek advice from members - will not tolerate disagreement with own opinion - manipulate members - dehumanizing, condescending, patronizing - believes nothing will happen unless he or she make it happen - does not have faith or trust in members - usually hostile and aggressive	- positive image of self and others - find meaning in others - sees self and others as becoming a person - assist others develop leadership qualities - accept weakness in self and others - flexible problem solving methods - highly motivated - promote participatory, supervisory & consultative leaders	- dislike control and structure - standard and rules are offensive to self - non-judgemental of others and self - accepts others as he is; friendly, warm and expect reciprocal relation - believes that self and others have the right to do their "own" thing
Functional Productivity	- members may be more efficient and productive but experience more hostility, competition, aggression - becomes less productive as time goes by due to low morale - more dependence and less creativity	- slower in getting productive but members are more strongly motivated - increased productivity with time - experienced teamwork and greater satisfaction with tasks - more creative	- less productive - spend time ineffectively - talk more about what to do - members become non-cooperative, bored and frustrated

Figure 3.1 Classical Styles of Leadership

GROUP DYNAMICS

Group dynamics is a term widely used in current literature and it refers to a complex interacting force that is happening in all groups at all times whether anyone is aware of it or not. Although the group has certain character, it is also dynamic, always moving and doing something. It changes, interacts, and reacts. The nature and direction of the movement is determined by forces being exerted on it from within the group itself and from the outside. Therefore, the interactions of these factors and their effects on a given group constitute its dynamics.

As members of the health team, nurses participate in many types of groups. Skills in group process and the role of the individual in groups will help develop sensitivity to the dynamics and help the group overcome problems and frustrations and move toward achievement of its goals. It will also assist nurses in developing acceptance for certain types of behaviors and, with practice, skills in dealing with the behavior in the group.

The knowledge of leadership and group structure will assist in the recognition of channels of communication and in working within the authority structure of the community health agencies. Leadership and group skills may prove a valuable tool in nursing practice since health care delivery involves a multitude of persons. It will alsp deepen one's understanding of the processes involved with groups of friends, family and community.

In sum, the factors that influence group dynamics may be drawn from infinite variety of sources and some of these may be simply stated as principles of group dynamics.

Some General Principles of Group Dynamics

1. The extent to which a group tends to be attractive to an individual and to command his or her loyalty depends on:
   a) the amount the group satisfies his or her needs and helps to achieve his or her goals
   b) provides acceptance and security
2. A person feels commited to a decision or goal to the extent that he or she has participated in determining it.
3. A group is an effective instrument for change and growth in individuals to the extent that:
   a) those to be changed and those who exert influence have a strong sense of belonging to the same group
   b) attraction of the group is greater than the discomfort of the change
   c) the members of the group share the perception that change is needed
   d) information relating to the need for change; plans for change and consequences of change is shared by all relevant people
   e) the group provides an opportunity for the individual to practice changed behavior without threat or punishment
   f) the individual is provided a means for measuring progress towards the changed goals.
4. Every force tends to induce an equal and opposite counterforce.
   i.e. The preferred strategy to accomplish change is the weakening of the forces resisting change rather than the addition of new positive forces toward change.
5. Every group is able to improve its ability to operate as a group to the extent that it consciously experiments with improved processes.
6. The better an individual understands the forces influencing his or her own behavior and that of the group, the better he or she will be able to contriubute constructively to the group and at the same time preserve his or her own integrity toward conformity and alienation.
7. The strength of pressure to conform is determined by:
   a) the strength of the attraction a group has for an individual
   b) the importance to the individual of the issue on which conformity is requested
   c) the degree of unanimity of the group toward required uniformity
8. The determinants of group effectiveness include:
   a) the extent to which a clear goal is present
   b) the degree to which the group goal mobilizes energies of group members behind group activities
   c) degree of agreement or conflict among the members concerning the means of obtaining a goal
   d) the degree of coordination of group activities and members
   e) the availability of needed resources—economic, material, legal, intellectual, etc.
   f) the degree of organization for the task
   g) the degree of appropriateness of the processes

GROUP EXPERIENCES IN PSYCHIATRY AND MENTAL HEALTH SETTINGS

The similarity of these processes among groups was recognized early in the history of group analysis and many efforts have been recorded and theorists have sought to identify and classify the steps common to all groups. While many believe in the similarities, other writers are not certain that their concepts are applicable to all groups and do not postulate a common process for all groups. It should be noted therefore, that while similarities in the developmental process exist, no one account can be taken as a prototype since each group will be different, depending on the nature of the group involved, its goal, theoretical orientation and personal needs of the members and style of leadership provided. For example, group processes utilized in growth and self-actualizing groups will place greater accent on emotional strength, limitation, liabilities of members; problems of self esteem; insight; development of new interpersonal and adaptation skills and so on. These will require greater depth and skills in the procedural operation and analysis of the group process as compared to a task-oriented group whose main focus is procedure-oriented to problem solve and/or meet a particular stated objective.

In psychiatric or mental health settings, the client does not usually see the group as meeting a need because many clients feel they do not need anything or if they feel a need, they want it satisfied by individual therapy. Furthermore, clients do not like other group members, and frequently dislike themselves and others who share their condition. Most clients participate in group experiences with great reluctance and misgivings. Conversely, in ordinary groups which are not therapy groups, people tend to get together to form a group and remain in the group because it satisfies some of their needs.

The concept of group dynamics continues to be the underlying basis for group activities utilized in psychiatry and mental health settings since the dynamics of the group itself set the motion of interactions and the group becomes a medium of treatment modality. It is obvious then that group experiences are dependent upon the skills of the nurse who is organizing and conducting group activities.

Objectives of Group Experiences for Clients

— allow practice of newly acquired or forgotten social skills

— an opportunity to solve specific problems or gain a different perspective on a problem

— a chance to release tension

— new experiences and learning

— change and diversion from daily living

— chance for mobility, status, recognition, achievement

— gives a sense of belonging and companionship

— learns to anticipate others' needs and vice-versa

— increase his/her self-understanding in relation to own needs, desires, conflicts and usual pattern of coping with life situations

Some Types of Group Activities

1. Remotivation Group: mainly utilized for long term, chronic, geriatric or retarded clients to encourage communication and sharing of experiences and interests, i.e. hygiene, current events, orientation, etc.
2. Recreational Groups: picnics, sight-seeing, sports and games
3. Social Groups: dances, talent shows, parties, sing-songs, etc.
4. Music Appreciation Groups: i.e. listening to variety of music followed by discussion and interpretation
5. Client Government group: client council meeting where a client is elected by other clients to act as chairperson and another client as recorder. Clients discuss any problems encountered in the unit and these are presented to staff members.
6. Problem-Solving Groups: discussion of domestic-vocational problems followed by solutions to the problem, i.e. how to apply for a job; how to look for housing, budgeting, etc.
7. Educational Groups: i.e. reading, learning and discussion
8. Arts and Crafts Group: often utilized as projective art techniques, i.e. painting, writing, drawing, leatherwork, pottery, weaving, etc.
9. Work Groups: i.e. gardens, laundry, kitchen, etc.
10. Role-Playing Groups: usually led by a highly skilled and trained staff member where a client is assigned to a situation in which he or she has formerly been unable to cope or has experienced conflict in coping with the situation.

Stalls in Group Process and Evaluation

Quite as important as the development of group process is that of becoming aware of the stalls that hinder the effectiveness of group work. It would be advisable for the reader to review the structure of the group and the variables affecting group dynamics stated earlier in this chapter as these are areas of knowledge that are essential in identifying the stalls that may affect the group process. Inherent in this frame of reference also includes the full use of understanding and the skill of working with groups that require an analysis of the stalls so that the group may progress toward its goals. Each dimension of a groups' life is related to and has an effect on other dimensions or other parts of the group. Thus, when there is a change in one dimension it will produce a strain on other dimensions. For example, a change in goals of the group, structure or behavior of members will affect other interrelated areas, and this may set up a chain reaction of problems and non-productivity.

Some common behaviors that hinder group effectiveness are:

1. *Blocking*—interfering with the progress of the group by introducing unrelated topics; arguing too much and rejecting the idea without consideration
2. *Fear of ridicule*—taking a stand which we fear will be unpopular to friends; fear of appearing ignorant; fear of deficiency in self expression
3. *Aggression*—attacking motives of others; criticizing or blaming others; deflating status of others
4. *Domination by others*—asserting authority in others; offers little or no encouragement; monopolizing member
5. *Withdrawal*—acting indifferently; being passive; doodling; whispering to others
6. *Seeking recognition*—calling attention to oneself by excessive talking; boisterous; presenting new unrelated ideas
7. *General feeling of inferiority*—lack of assertive skills; fear of being contradicted; fear of offending others; fear of disclosing self

Evaluation of Group Process

A. *Considerations for the effectiveness of group action:*
   1. Do the goals that we have established for each meeting help us to reach our goals?
   2. Do we plan our meetings in relation to our objectives? Does one person take this responsibility or do all the members share in it?
   3. Do we clarify the meaning of our goals and procedures whenever necessary during the meetings?
   4. Do we summarize our progress from time to time?
   5. Do we use suitable methods of procedure?
   6. Do we evaluate the efficiency of our methods of functioning?
   7. Do we watch our discussion to see if we understand each other?
   8. Do we spread responsibility throughout the group?
   9. Do we have an atmosphere in which all are free to express ideas and feelings?
   10. Do we exhibit a feeling or responsibility to restrict our contributions to those which are helpful to the group?

B. *Considerations of self in the group:*
   1. What part did I play in this group discussion?
      Was I an active participant?
      Was I an active listener to the contributions of others?
      Did I dominate the group?
      Did I stray from the point under discussion?
      Was I timid about expressing my point of view?
   2. Was I well prepared to participate in the group discussion?
      Did I do the necessary reading for this discussion?
      Did I select and organize my facts in such a way as to make an interesting presentation to the group?

Did I support my view with relevant facts?

Did I find questions unanswered in my mind because of insufficient data?

Did I use reliable sources of information for the facts I needed?

3. What was my attitude during the group discussion?

Was I opinionated?

Was I willing to respect the point of view held by other group members?

Was I willing to weigh the varying points of view presented before arriving at a final conclusion?

Was I too willing to compromise on issues I regarded as important?

Was I eager to hear what other members of the group were thinking?

4. Did I benefit from participating in this group discussion?

Did I do clear thinking or did I merely rearrange my prejudices?

Will the skills I acquired in the group discussion help me to think clearly and intelligently in new situations?

C. *Consideration of leadership role:*

1. Who emerged as a leader in the group?
2. What type of leadership was provided?
3. How did the members feel toward the leader?

Suggested Readings

Benne, K. D. and Sheats, P., *Functional Roles of Group Members.* Journal of Social Issues 4:41–49–1948

Bonner, H., *Group Dynamics: Principles and Applications.* New York. Ronald Press. 1964

Cartwright, D., and Zander, A., *Group Dynamics: Research and Theory.* New York. Harper and Row Publishers. 1968

Clark, C. C., *The Nurse as Group Leader.* New York. Springer Publishing Co., 1977

Klein, J., *The Study of Groups.* The International Library of Sociology and Social Reconstruction. London. Routledge and Kogan Paul Ltd., 1965

Knowles, M. and Knowles, H., *Introduction to Group Process.* New York. Association Press, 1959

Kreigh, H. and Perko, J. *Psychiatric and Mental Health Nursing: Commitment to Care and Concern.* 2nd ed. Reston, Virginia. Reston Publishing Co., A Prentice Hall Co., 1983

Lewin, K., *Field Theory in Social Service.* D. Cartwright Ed. New York. Harper and Brothers. 1951

Marram, G. D., *The Group Approach in Nursing Practice.* St. Louis. The C. V. Mosby Co., 1973

Whitaker, D. S., *A Group Centered Approach.* Group Process 7:37–57–1967

Yalom, I., *The Theory and Practice of Group Psychotherapy.* New York. Basic Books Inc. Publishers, 1971

Exercise 12

GROUP PROCESS I

Duration: 20 minutes

Directions: 1. Participants divide into two (2) groups of 8–10, forming a small inner circle; an outer group circle of 8–10 participants who will act as observer of the group process.

2. The inner circle will be given the series of aspirations stated below to which the participants will choose the three (3) most important items to him or her.

3. At the conclusion of 20 minutes, the inner circle group should have a consensus of the three (3) important items that are acceptable to each member.

Aspirations:

a. To set your own working conditions
b. To become a millionaire
c. To master the profession of your choice
d. To be famous, respected and admired
e. To be the most attractive person
f. To have a perfect marriage
g. To have lots of friends
h. To travel and see the world
i. To have peace in the world
j. To be healthy and happy

4. The participants of the inner circle are asked the following questions after the group has decided about the three most important aspirations.
a. How understood and listened to did you feel in the group?
b. How much influence do you feel you had on the group's decision?
c. How responsible and committed do you feel about the decision?
d. How satisfied are you with your group's performance?
e. State three objectives describing the way you feel now.

5. Outer group circle participants will watch the inner circle group at work and make note of the behaviors displayed by each member; observe the functional roles assumed by members; assess the social climate of the group process.

6. *Post discussion*
Both groups share and discuss their own experiences and observation of the group process.

Exercise 13

GROUP PROCESS II

Duration: 20 minutes

Directions: 1. Repeat the procedure of Exercise 12 with the exception of the list of aspirations to be discussed. In other words, the inner circle group will have no tasks assigned and it is up to the participants to decide on what topics each member wishes to discuss.

2. *Post-discussion*
   a) Are there differences and similarities in the group process?
   b) How are the roles allocated?
   c) How did the discussion work? Was it emotional or objective?
   d) Did all participants become involved?
   e) How did the participants make their decision?
   f) How did the participants feel?

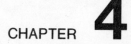

Psychosocial Assessment

-Physiological Mode
-Self-Concept Mode
-Role Function Mode
-Interdependence Mode

Psychosocial assessment presupposes an understanding of human behavior. Growth and development, communication skills and interaction process since these areas of knowledge are essential in the formulation of care.

People do not behave in certain ways for no reason at all and there is always something behind it all to make them act the way they do. Thus, "every behavior has a meaning" and if our goal is to understand the client, it is useless to focus our attention upon certain parts or aspects of the client's behavior. Human beings are not made of separate physical and psychosocial entity; instead, the two form a unit and function as one. Nurses, therefore, need to focus on the client as a whole.

Contrary to the myth of clients being embarrassed by enquiries about human relations, sexual function and life style, very often clients are willing and eager to express their concerns and views on questions being asked. The nurse may be uncomfortable and embarrassed but the client seldom is. If the client becomes hesitant in answering questions he or she has usually sensed the nurse's own discomfort. As long as the client views the nurse as a potential source of help, he or she will communicate more or less freely any material that the client may feel pertinent to the problem.

Another misconception is the belief that psychosocial assessment is only relevant to psychiatric clients and that it is unnecessary to bother with psychosocial assessment on a client who is undergoing surgery or for a client who is suffering from a medical condition.

The model of psychosocial assessment stated in this manual is arranged under various sections to provide the learner with a scheme to organize his or her observation during the assessment process. According to this model, man is viewed as a psychosocial being who is in constant interaction with a changing environment, and man in his attempt to cope with internal and external changes, adapts to the stimuli in four different dimensions—physiological, self-concept, role function, and interdependence modes, which may be adaptive or maladaptive. This view necessitates looking at behaviors within the individual and his total responses to a given stimuli as well as at the process of adaptation. Rather than thinking about the signs and symptoms of a given condition or disease, it is necessary to analyze the condition according to these four modes of adaptation, since each of these modes is interrelated and interacts with one another to preserve and maintain physiological, psychological and social integrity. For example, the physiological modes include needs such as sleep, exercise, rest, nutrition, elimination, electrolytes, oxygen, and so on; while the self-concept mode encompasses the need for psychological integrity and includes anxiety, depression, guilt, powerlessness, body image problems, alteration or disturbances of thinking process. Role function and interdependence behaviors are related to social integrity and explore man's diversified roles in the environment, his needs for belonging and achievement, dependency and independence.

PHYSIOLOGICAL MODE

As one studies the concept of homeostasis, one can readily see that adaptation at all levels may be viewed from the point of homeostasis as the individual attempts to maintain a certain balance due to constant dealing with the internal and external changes in the environment. Because of this, a system may experience alteration in responses and adapt to the stimuli in various modes which involve a need for change if the individual is to deal with the stressful situation and promote the healing process.

The investigation and establishment of physiological baseline responses is a technical part of psychosocial assessment to determine adaptive and maladaptive functioning of the body and the correlation of emotional factors to physical symptoms which have been the subject of stress related conditions.

The areas to be explored and described under this mode are:

- exercise and rest, i.e. sleep patterns and activities
- nutrition, i.e. anorexia, nutritional status, nausea and vomiting
- elimination, i.e. constipation, diarrhea, incontinence, perspiration
- fluid and electrolyte, i.e. edema, dehydration, level of consciousness
- oxygen and circulation, i.e. respiration, hypoxia, dyspnea, respiratory failure and shock
- temperature, i.e. fever, cold
- senses, i.e. blindness, deafness, sensory deprivation, anasthesia
- safety, i.e. injury to tissue

SELF-CONCEPT MODE

The importance of self concept in meeting the needs of client goes far beyond providing the basis of care because self concept exerts powerful influence on every aspect of human behavior and it is what makes each individual unique and different from others.

The self concept of the client is the frame of reference from which observations can be made to understand the needs and predict the client's behavior. Self concept include all those aspects of perceptions to which a person refers to the "I" or "Me" of the physical self; the organization of ideas, beliefs and values that the person places upon the various qualities of the personal self which is manifested in ethical-moral, consistency and ideal expectations of oneself.

The perpetuating effect of self concept is by no means limiting and it operates on both the adaptive and maladaptive levels. People with positive self concept will likely behave with confidence and the existence of such high self-esteem will create stability and cause others to react in a similar fashion. Negative self concept, on the other hand, will lead to maladaptive behaviors as commonly manifested in clients with emotional and psychiatric problems.

When the nurse knows how client perceives himself or herself, much of the behavior becomes understandable and the helper can predict with some accuracy what the client will likely do next and the nurse will be able to assess, plan and implement appropriate nursing interventions.

The outline for organizing data to explore self-concept is:

a. General Appearance
   - detailed description of the client, i.e. body build, complexion
   - personal hygiene and grooming, i.e. dishevelled look, inappropriate grooming, meticulousness
   - facial expression, i.e. angry, tearful
   - body language, i.e. posture, movement
b. Method of Communication
   - physical qualities of voice, i.e. soft, loud, monotone
   - flow of speech, i.e. talkative, repetitive, monosyllabic
   - motor behavior, i.e. fidgeting, pacing, wringing of hands, posture

c. Affect or Feeling Tone
- emotion expressed such as sadness, hostility, euphoria, guilt, powerlessness and so forth.
If the emotions expressed are obvious, it is important to focus on what led to the feeling that the client is experiencing at the time and it is significant to determine the following areas:
- is the client aware of these feelings
- how are these feelings being handled
- is the client able to identify the cause of these feelings

d. Mental State
Though processes can be observed in terms of:
- content, i.e. delusion, suicidal thoughts, phobias
- progression, i.e. flight of ideas, circumstantiality
- perception, i.e. hallucinations, suspiciousness
- intellectual functions, i.e. preoccupation, poor concentration, misinterpretation, impaired judgment, disorientation

e. Ego Assessment
- type of defense mechanisms utilized
- does the client see self as needing help
- does the client observe any changes in his own behavior
- presence of healthy attributes, i.e. talents, skills, self-care, effective coping skills

ROLE FUNCTION MODE

The concept of role function is significant in understanding the client, his or her interaction with others and the context in which the behavior occurs since the individual's self concept and roles are developed through these interactions. In other words, a role is a set of regulated norms specifying a pattern of behavior in a specified situation and the person's role conception is influenced by variety of factors such as occupation, social class, significant others, culture, life style, social network, and the like. The way an individual will enact role will depend upon the person's conceptualization of the role and influence of the self system. Roles are dynamic in the sense that the person's role relationship and expectation can change due to transition in growth and development, health-illness continuum and situations.

The role function of the client must be employed as a baseline date in assessing, planning and implementing. Each client has numerous positions which can be ascribed—those positions usually determined by age, sex, and culture; and those achieved positions which are acquired through the individual's accomplishment. The position of being a client is only one of the many positions that the client occupies and by becoming aware of this the nurse will be cognizant of the social network that may influence the client's responses to interventions; will facilitate adaptation by assisting the client identify potential role transitions and incorporate the new changed role into self esteem, thus preventing role failure and role conflict.

Concomitant with role function is the level of motivation of the client to either resume or relinquish that particular role and the likelihood of improvement will be influenced by this aspiration and may also provide clues to the problems and conflict involved.

In exploring the area of role function, it is important to assess the client according to the following:

- ascribed role, i.e. age, sex, culture

- achieved role, i.e. parental, siblings, occupation, profession and the like

- attitude toward role

- attitude toward role changes and transition

- level of motivation

- patterns of role enactment

- evidence of role failure and conflict

INTERDEPENDENCE MODE

The development of behavior is not determined solely by heredity, maturation or culture into which an individual is born. Some of the knowledge acquired about self are discovered through interactions with others and the physical world. From these experiences, dependency or the need to depend on others for fulfillment of physiological and psychological needs begins with birth and continues until one is fully grown and becomes independent. Most behavior is of a definite nature and is in response to a need that a person is fully aware of and which causes the person to act to fill these needs. With maturity, more important to the growth of self are the need for affiliation which are implied by the desire for social acceptance and the need to achieve, the continuous search for fulfillment and enhancement. The process of changing from dependency to independency is not an easy one but rather is one marked by many conflicts and desires to remain in the dependent role. There is no such state of complete independence. In our present society, growing more complex daily, individuals are increasingly becoming more inter-dependent on others for fulfillment of psychosocial needs such as love, affection and companionship. Well, adaptive persons will make the necessary compromise between dependent and independent role and is capable of making that decision as well. A maladaptive person will have difficulty balancing and coping with changes and will employ instead a series of maladaptive behaviors.

Other issues involved in assessing the interdependency mode is the support system of the client, past and present relation with family and other significant figures so that attempts will be made to re-establish such interdependency. In order to accomplish this, the nurse should determine the presence or absence of interdependency by focusing on the following:

- client's feelings about family, significant others, peers and other people
- influence of the "perceived" support over the client's life
- effect of illness on family and their reaction
- influence of family on client
- how client feels and relates in social and working situation
- the life style of client

Suggested Readings

Clark, C., *Nursing Concepts and Processes.* Albany, New York. Delmar Publishers, 1977

Kolb, L. C., *Noyes' Modern Clinical Psychiary,* 10th ed., Philadelphia. W. B. Saunders Co., 1982

Kreigh, H. and Perko, J. E., *Psychiatric and Mental Health Nursing, Commitment to Care and Concern,* 2nd ed., Reston, Virginia. Reston Publishing Co. Inc., 1983

Randall, B., et al., *Adaptation Nursing—The Roy Conceptual Model Applied,* St. Louis. The C. V. Mosby Co., 1982

Roy, Sister Callista, *Introduction to Nursing: An Adaptation Model.* Englewood Cliffs, New Jersey. Prentice Hall Inc., 1976

Stuart, G. W. and Sundeen, S. J., *Principles and Practice of Psychiatric Nursing,* 2nd ed., St. Louis. The C. V. Mosby Co., 1983

Exercise 14

PSYCHOSOCIAL ASSESSMENT I

Duration: 10 minutes

Direction: Ask two participants to role play an assessment interview. One participant will play the role of the nurse, the other participant will act in the role of the client, attempting to display all the elements or content areas of psychosocial assessment.

The rest of the class will observe the following:

– communication techniques utilized
– verbal and non-verbal behavior of both participants
– identify the factors that hinder or facilitate the interview process

After the interview, have both participants express how they felt in the role that they have assumed according to:

– physiological mode

– self concept mode

– role function mode

– interdepedence mode

Exercise 15
VOCABULARY

Make a list of at least five (5) adjectives that will describe the following behaviors.

Behaviors   *Adjectives*

1. Facial expression   _____

2. Speech   _____

3. Posture   _____

4. Motor activity   _____

5. Affect or mood   _____

6. Thoughts   _____

7. Personal grooming   _____

8. Eating habits   _____

9. Elimination habits   _____

10. Sleep habits   _____

Exercise 16

PSYCHOSOCIAL ASSESSMENT II

Duration: 10 minutes

Direction: Match the psychosocial assessment areas in Column I with appropriate questionings in Column II to reflect the nurse's intent in the assessment process, and in Column III to reflect the client's statement of his or her status.

Column I

a. physiological mode
b. self-concept mode
c. role function mode
d. interdependence mode

Column II—Nurse's Questions

_____ 1. How does your family feel about you not being able to work?

_____ 2. How did you sleep last night?

_____ 3. Are you thinking of killing yourself?

_____ 4. What do you do to relieve your tensions?

_____ 5. Who can you depend on to help you?

_____ 6. What do you think is happening to you right now?

_____ 7. How does it feel to be in the hospital as a client?

_____ 8. Do you have any physical symptoms since you felt upset?

_____ 9. How does your illness affect your status in your family?

_____ 10. Do you have any interests that you can do while being a client?

Column III—Client's Statements

_____ 1. I have difficulty breathing, I cannot eat or sleep.

_____ 2. I am quite capable of looking after myself.

_____ 3. Who will look after my family when I am ill?

_____ 4. Sometimes I feel like ending it all.

_____ 5. My boss at work is not too happy with me being ill frequently.

_____ 6. I feel so helpless and losing control of the situation.

_____ 7. I cannot seem to do well in everything I do.

_____ 8. Perhaps I can read to avoid boredom in the hospital.

_____ 9. I used to jog and exercise when I felt tense.

_____ 10. People at work couldn't care less.

Exercise 17

MALADAPTIVE BEHAVIOR WORKSHEET

Duration: Relate to client assignments

Direction: As defined

Disorders of Perception	Definition	Identify the Disorder in a Nursing Situation and Related Psychopathology
1) Illusion		
2) Hallucination Types – Auditory – Visual – Tactile – Olfactory – Gustatory		

Disorders of Thinking	Definition	Identify the Disorder in a Nursing Situation and Related Psychopathology
1) Autism		

Disorders of Thinking	Definition	Identify the Disorder in a Nursing Situation and Related Psychopathology

2) Delusion
   Types
   – Grandeur
   – Persecution
   – Omnipotence
   – Nihilistic
   – Somatic		

3) Ideas of Reference		
4) Obsession		
5) Phobia		

Disorders of Thinking	Definition	Identify the Disorder in a Nursing Situation and Related Psychopathology
6) Flight of Ideas		
7) Circumstantiality		
8) Incoherence		
9) Blocking		

Disorders of Thinking	Definition	Identify the Disorder in a Nursing Situation and Related Psychopathology
10) Suggestibility		

Disorders of Consciousness	Definition	Identify the Disorder in a Nursing Situation and Related Psychopathology
1) Confusion		
2) Stupor		

Disorders of Consciousness	Definition	Identify the Disorder in a Nursing Situation and Related Psychopathology
3) Delirium		
4) Disorientation		

Disorders of Affect	Definition	Identify the Disorder in a Nursing Situation and Related Psychopathology
1) Apathy		

Disorders of Affect	Definition	Identify the Disorder in a Nursing Situation and Related Psychopathology
2) Passivity		
3) Lethargy		
4) Labile Mood		

Disorders of Memory	Definition	Identify the Disorder in a Nursing Situation and Related Psychopathology

1) Amnesia
Types
  – Antrograde
  – Retrograde		

2) Confabulation		
3) Retrospective Falsification		

Disorders of Motor Activity	Definition	Identify the Disorder in a Nursing Situation and Related Psychopathology
1) Stereotype Behaviour		
2) Catalepsy		
3) Mannerism		
4) Compulsion		

Disorders of Motor Activity	Definition	Identify the Disorder in a Nursing Situation and Related Psychopathology
5) Retardation		
6) Echopraxia		

Disorders of Speech	Definition	Identify the Disorder in a Nursing Situation and Related Psychopathology
1) Echolalia		

Disorders of Speech	Definition	Identify the Disorder in a Nursing Situation and Related Psychopathology
2) Neologism		
3) Clang Association		

CHAPTER 5

Mental Health Concepts

- Anxiety
- Anger and Hostility
- Loss
- Guilt
- Powerlessness
- Loneliness

Mental health concepts are clusters of ideas, propositions and behavioral responses pertaining to man's emotional, mental and social state. Although people have some idea of what emotions are, most would be hard pressed to define them because emotion is a complex behavioral response involving physiological and psychological interactions. It is commonly best described by providing a number of emotional states or emotional situations that one is experiencing or has experienced. Love, hate, anger, hostility, loss, guilt, powerlessness, excitement and enjoyment are only a few emotions that describe feelings that many people experience to some degree on a daily basis.

The capacity to feel is as much a part of being a person as is the capacity to think and reason. One can rationalize it is natural to have emotions and yet one may commonly feel that these feelings are disruptive, a source of difficulty and discontentment in life. Although emotions are spontaneous reactions to factors over which individuals have little control, it is not the feelings that are the source of problems, but the way a person deals with them.

Physiologically, there are changes in both muscular and glandular activities which generally produce marked change in normal functions. Psychologically, shifts in expressions of emotions and maladaptive behaviors becomes quite evident.

It is in the process of dealing with emotions that health professionals will find the key to understand the client. Under the stress that is thus produced, inner feelings, conflicts and breakdown of ego defenses are more likely to be expressed.

Historically speaking, psychiatric nursing gained its recognition as a nursing specialty by process of differentiation from other aspects of nursing. As a reaction to the increasing recognition and implementation of holistic approach to client care, other areas of nursing practice are more and more infiltrated by concepts originating from psychopathology, other behavioral sciences and psychiatric nursing skills.

Its main impetus came from the growing awareness of the need of how to deal with maladaptive responses of clients to being physically ill as well as how to deal with the emotional problems that contribute to their being ill outside the classical psychiatric boundaries.

Clinicians are becoming more cognizant of the fact that a purely physical and impersonal approach to clients is quite inadequate. To a certain extent, mental hygiene can be looked at as an aspect of general hygiene.

In these circumstances, it is not surprising that there is a greater trend and utilization of psychiatric nursing knowledge and techniques in everyday nursing practice. It can hardly be doubted that this not only contributes significantly to the well-being of the client as a person, but it also helps society develop a solid health-promoting basis in mental health.

The following mental health concepts selected for this Manual are behavioral responses that nurses need to know and acquire in order to meet and promote emotional health of clients in any given setting. Understanding the concepts that help explain the behavior will lead to expected outcomes. It is also imperative that the student apply these concepts to his/her ownself so that he or she may fully understand what the client is experiencing and vice-versa.

CONCEPT OF ANXIETY

Anxiety is a universal emotional phenomenon experienced by all at some time or another. Most people of all ages, both healthy and mentally ill, strive to ward off anxiety or to keep it from awareness because of its unpleasantness. It is one of the most commonly and loosely used terms in psychiatry and confusion has resulted from gradual changes in the emphasis of its meaning. Emotionally ill clients attempt to dispel anxiety by developing mental symptoms. The role of anxiety in psychopathology will be described further according to various psychiatric conditions in subsequent chapters. The well adjusted individual attempts to counteract anxiety by mobilization of the energy into constructive channels. One of the difficulties with the concept of anxiety is the necessity to differentiate it from fear. While this differentiation is not always easy or even possible at times, fear is a relatively well defined response to real or imagined danger, and anxiety is more likely to be vague, diffuse and undefined. Fear is a learned reaction to external events. Anxiety, a more chronic state, is usually produced by the conditioning of physiological reactions.

The differentiation between normal and pathological anxiety is important. The determining factors which assist in establishing whether the anxiety reaction is normal or pathological are the intensity and duration of the emotional state and objective validity of precipitating events. For example, when a person has been told that a biopsy has revealed the presence of malignant tissue, the individual could be expected to display a great deal of anxiety. This should be viewed as a normal reaction to a very stressful event.

New and unknown situations can create anxiety in normal well adjusted individuals. Hospitalization may be classified as an anxiety-producer and there are many factors present which tend to create apprehension in those who are hospitalized. They have been removed from their normal routine, they are not physically well and may tend to be weak and vulnerable. Their normal support system of friends and relatives has been at least partially replaced.

Finally, the individual finds himself or herself in a situation which is foreign and one which most people do not understand. The possibility of medical complications or potential discovery of more serious problems will tend to add to the general feeling of discomfort and apprehension. Anxiety, then, may be described as a state of persistent, diffuse feeling of dread, apprehension, unpleasant uneasiness and impending doom.

Essential Aspects of Anxiety

- It is an energy and as such, it cannot be observed directly. Therefore it can only be inferred from the relief behavior that occurs; for example, fight and flight behaviors.
- It is an emotion without specific identifiable cause or it may be that the emotion may be displaced from its original source unconsciously.
- It is a psychophysiological response.
- It is a response to threat, whether real or imaginary.
- It is a universal emotional experience.
- It has a constructive and destructive aspect.
- It is a symptom in almost any psychiatric syndrome.
- It is communicated interpersonally.
- It plays a major role in the dynamics of personality organization and disorganization. First as a signal that alerts one to impending danger enabling the person to set in motion the defensive and adjustive process which will serve to protect the person against inner threats; secondly, as a symptom which is expressed in the breakdown of defenses in the personality. In this role, anxiety becomes the basic symptom in a number of psychiatric disturbances as mentioned above.

Operational Definition of Anxiety

Some discussion of a working definition of the concept of anxiety is necessary since anxiety is frequently manifested in the behavior of the individual and to furnish the practitioner with tools that will enable him or her to deal with the phenomenon of anxiety. Operationally, when the individual's basic needs and expectations are not met, anxiety occurs. Initially, the person has some expectations and needs which may be conscious or unconscious and these expectations are the result of his or her past experiences with significant others. The individual then attempts and anticipates fulfillment of these expectations. If expectations are not met, either by the individual himself or by others in the environment, the person will become powerless, anxious and will experience a sense of loss at this time. The energy is then mobilized through the utilization of automatic responses as a means of coping with the anxiety as a temporary relief. The pattern of relief behavior that an individual utilizes varies from person to person. A previous learned pattern of adjustment, whether appropriate or inappropriate to the immediate situation, will be maintained and perceived by the person as the real and valid coping mechanisms; for example, anger, inhibition, withdrawal, somatization, aggression, and so forth, and quite often the individual will rationalize and justify his relief behavior in an attempt to preserve and maintain the integrity of his ego. Thus, the needs and expectations are not gratified, the pattern does not change, the cycle becomes repetitive and the person continues to feel anxious.

Anxiety State in Childhood

Although anxiety state in childhood is similar to that of an adult where anxiety arises as a response to a given threat, the threats are more complex, varied, and include especially those associated with biological maturation and family life. Furthermore, the child is less able to discern the cause of the threat and the signs of anxiety are often given by parents or significant others. Fearfulness and unhappiness are quite often displayed whenever the child is faced with new situations and behavior problems ensue.

The fears of a child shift with age. A newborn is alarmed by loud noises and loss of support and by about six months, the child may cry with anxiety if approached by strangers. After the age of one year, there is the realization of his or her full dependency on the mother figure for comfort and security and they are apt to become more suspicious of strangers. When his or her need for security is satisfied, the child may strive for some independent action and exploration for a short time and immediately returns to the mother figure for comfort and safety.

Increased dependency on the mother figure tends to become more pronounced between the ages of two or three. The child displays extreme shyness with strangers, takes a longer time to feel at ease in a group situation and is reluctant to being left alone, especially at bedtime and is extremely sensitive to any sudden or prolonged separation. Anxiety about wetting often seems to play a part in anxieties of childhood. It may appear that the child's wetting is associated with his or her fear that it will displease the mother and is perceived as the reason for the mother's leaving.

The anxieties of a child by the age of three or four are more complex as the child has reached a stage of mental and emotional development where he or she can imagine and apply dangers to themselves which they never experienced. For example, the child may acquire some specific fears, such as fear of objects, strangers, social and school situations, bodily differences, any form of disability or even death. Changes in appetite and sleep disturbances may emerge. Nocturnal anxieties associated with frequent awakening, screaming and enuresis may be displayed. These are by-products of various stages of emotional development and if not properly handled may lead to a more serious problem in later life.

Levels of Anxiety

The degree of anxiety is characterized by a typical state of awareness, performance, ability to concentrate and focus on what is really happening and the successful or unsuccessful method of coping with anxiety.

It is important to note the constructive aspect of anxiety in that anxiety may act as a drive to overcome behavior, eliminate and resolve a threat. It has been shown that there is an optimal level of anxiety drive in human beings which is responsible for proficient performance and productivity. Anxiety also evokes behavioral responses which is anxiety reducing and restores homeostasis.

Mild Level of Anxiety (≁) Learning State:

- perception is alert and keen. Perceptual field is broad and the individual is able to focus on what is really happening
- is able to discuss and talk about the situation, own feelings, thoughts, actions
- is able to analyze situations, interpret and make connections
- is able to perceive the situation in relation to the total event
- concentrates all energy for intense activity and proficient performance
- increased physiological functioning

Moderate Level of Anxiety (≁≁)

- perceptual field becomes narrow and there is limited ability to concentrate and focus on what is really happening
- may focus on certain subjects or details of the events and concentrate on this topic
- events cannot be seen in relation to other situations
- may experience free-floating anxiety, feelings of impending doom, may attach these feelings to any objects to explain the feelings of discomfort

Severe Level of Anxiety (≁≁≁)

- perceptual field is greatly reduced and is handicapping
- focuses on irrelevant details of the events which becomes disturbed
- has difficulty hearing, seeing and is unable to make logical connections on what is actually happening
- may become paralyzed in thoughts and actions

Panic Level of Anxiety (≁≁≁≁)

- details of the events are distorted, forgotten or exaggerated
- unable to communicate, communication may be blocked, irrelevant, has no connection or logical understanding of what is being discussed
- feels helpless, powerless, awe, dread, terror
- mobilizes energy into anger, becomes assaultive, destructive or escapes completely
- total disorganization of personality

Causes of Anxiety

Causes then of anxiety may be summed up as follows: any threat to the psychobiological equilibrium of an individual will produce anxiety and such threats may fall into the following categories, namely:

1. *Biological Threat*
   - any threat to the tendency of an individual to maintain normal body functioning, i.e., temperature control, vasomotor stability, etc.
   - any threat that produces alterations in homeostatic process which may result from illness, trauma and irreversible pathology
2. *Psychological Threat*
   - any threat to the innate energy of the individual to maintain the established views of oneself, self-concept, and set patterns of values and expectations
3. *Social Threat*
   - any threat to role change and status, sense of belonging and loss of freedom
4. *Spiritual Threat*
   - any threat to one's own beliefs, moral standards

Behavioral Manifestation of Anxiety

Anxiety has been labelled the most basic emotion because of its roots in the behavior of lower animals where it acts as primitive generalized response to a threat. Under the threat of danger, animals usually display one or two reactions, the flight or fight responses. In either case, a complex physiological reaction prepares the animal so that it is better equipped to deal with danger. The release of the hormone adrenalin, by the adrenal glands, is one of the physiological changes which accompany anxiety. Imbalance of the sympathetic and parasympathetic activity is responsible for many of the somatic concomitants of anxiety. While lower animals are primarily threatened by external environmental dangers, people are also threatened by internal stimuli such as thought, feelings, and impulses. Therefore, anxiety can be present in human beings even when there is no discernible threat apparent to the observer. The following table will demonstrate the behavioral manifestation of anxiety for assessment purposes according to physiological, self-concept, role function and interdependence modes.

ASSESSMENT
BEHAVIORAL MANIFESTATION OF ANXIETY

Physiological Mode	Self-Concept Mode	Role Function Mode	Interdependence Mode
– changes in skin turgor, extreme shift in body temperature, perspiration, cold clammy skin, pale appearance, dry mouth, skin rash	– irritableness – weepiness – anger – guilt – critical of self and others	– feelings of helplessness – feelings of powerlessness – feelings of loss – poor judgement	– quarrelsomeness – oversolicitousness – demanding – compliant – alienation
– changes in pupillary reactions, increased pulse rate, heart rate and respiration, increased blood pressure, headaches	– reduced interest – interferences with thinking process – poor concentration – distorted perception	– indecisiveness – seeking constant reassurance – distorted perception	– isolation – dependent – negativism – critical of others
– muscular tension, tremors; restlessness, fidgety, hyperactivity, muscle spasm	– feelings of worthlessness – diminished mental acuity	– negativism – preoccupation	– aggression
– diarrhea, constipation, polyuria, flatulence	– selective inattention – inability to relate		
– sensation of lump in the throat, abdominal "churning," chest pain and hyperventilation syndrome			
– changes in eating habits such as polyphagia, anorexia, nausea and vomiting			

How we feel when under anxiety

Physiological Mode	Self-Concept Mode	Role Function Mode	Interdependence Mode
– changes in sleep patterns from insomnia or somnolence – stuttering, tics – gastrointestinal disturbances such as peptic ulcers, chronic ulcerative colitis – amenorrhea			

PLANNING AND IMPLEMENTATION

Strategies	Rationale
Physiological Mode – Simulate as closely as possible previous healthy habits of eating, elimination, sleep patterns and activities	– physiological manifestation of anxiety will increase feeling of discomfort, distresss and threat – maintenance of familiar activities of daily living will prevent undue increase in anxiety – allay anxieties of loss of control of oneself – to promote and maintain physiological functions
Self-Concept Mode – Validate your observations with client	– to indicate awareness of what he or she is experiencing – to evaluate behaviors manifested. Client's responses to anxiety can be misleading – anxiety tends to increase if unrecognized and unattended
– Assist client to identify feelings	– to ascertain verbal and nonverbal cues and note any inconsistencies – to assist client to relate feelings to the term "anxiety" – to determine client's accuracy of perception – to provide outlet and release of mounting distress – to determine if anxiety is normal or pathological – to assist client to relate and express what is happening as opposed to his or her expectations
– Stay with client	– to convey attitude of interest in reduction of anxiety. Client experiences extreme feelings of fearfulness, loss of control and may become panicked; may react negatively as a result of frustrations – to establish rapport – presence of others and staff will provide reassurance and feeling of safety – to provide an accepting and non-judgmental environment – to provide opportunity to initiate connections and establish rapport

Strategies	Rationale
– Evaluate sources of anxiety	– to assist client to identify the cause of anxiety
	– to determine whether the source of anxiety is biological, social, psychological or environmental
	– ascertain if threat is real or imaginary
	– to clarify sequence of events related to present anxiety
– Explore previous coping methods for relief	– to assist client to become aware of his or her coping behavior
	– to offer opportunities to develop alternative ways of coping
	– to assist client to gain new perspective of the situation
Role Function Mode	
– Orientate to new surroundings, treatment plan and routine activities	– to allay feelings of uncertainty
	– to promote sense of control
	– to maintain feelings of independence
	– to prevent feelings of alienation
	– to ensure participation and effectiveness of treatment plan
	– Activities not familiar will induce further anxiety
– Provide opportunity to work on own problems at own pace	– to maintain self-esteem and independence on problem-solving skills
	– to facilitate previous level of healthy functioning
Interdependence Mode	
– Determine client's need for medication	– to inform other health team members
	– to provide relief from distress
	– to prevent mounting of anxiety level
– Inform team members of the client's pathological responses to anxiety	– behavioral responses may indicate severe underlying conflicts which may necessitate psychiatric referral
– Involve support system in treatment plan	– to foster trust and co-operativeness in health team members
	– to ensure effectiveness of care and treatment

Evaluation
- Assess response of client to treatment plan
- Evaluate effectiveness of nursing interventions
- Modify plan of care according to changing needs of the client
- Re-assessment of the goals of plan of care
- Share and collaborate with other team members the revision of plan

ANXIETY

depends how they sta

Situation 1

The coordinator of the Nursing Program left you a note stating "I would like to see you as soon as your class is over. It is of great importance that we discuss your academic standing in the program. Please see my secretary for an appointment."

1) List and describe your responses to the above situation according to:

    a. physiological mode

    can't concentrate, ↑ H.R. , sweaty palms
    nauseated, stomach hurt,

    b. self-concept mode
    esteem
    failure

    c. role function mode
    as a student
    student seeing major director

    d. interdependence mode
    dependent?
    reach out for a friend

2) Identify some of the relief behaviors that you have utilized as means of coping with the above situation.

Situation II

1) You appear to have difficulty developing manual dexterity in giving intramuscular injections. This is the third time you have failed your skill performance test.
    During preparation and administration of the injection, identify and describe your ability to:

    – observe, listen and follow instructions

    – focus attention

– learn

– function

2) Identify your coping behavior and state whether it is a successful or unsuccessful method of handling your anxiety.

Situation III

Your patient, Mrs. Smith, a 70 year old female, is quite demanding and critical of the nursing staff on the medical unit to which you are assigned. Mrs. Smith absolutely refuses to have a student nurse assigned to her and states, "I do not wish to be a guinea pig."

1) How would you react to Mrs. Smith while attending to her needs and how did you behave?

2) How would you handle the situation?

3) What are the possible reasons for Mrs. Smith's behavior?

Situation IV

Jamie, a 5 year old boy, was admitted to the hospital for tonsillectomy.

1) What behavioral manifestation will be displayed by Jamie to indicate anxiety?

2) What nursing actions will you implement to reduce Jamie's anxiety?

Situation V

Mrs. V., a 36 year old divorced female patient and mother of two children, is scheduled for hysterectomy at 1200 hours. While awaiting her pre-operative medication, you noted Mrs. V. is sitting by the window, looking out with a sad, worried look on her face. When approached, Mrs. V. was pleased to see you, was overly pleasant and co-operative when instructed to use the hospital gown and get back to bed. Her skin is cold to touch, she asked you a few times the exact hour of surgery and stated that when her sister had the same operation, she developed some complications. You further observed that Mrs. V. has been to the washroom twice during the short time that you were with her.

1) List and describe the adaptive responses of Mrs. V. to anxiety according to:

   a) physiological mode

   ↑ urination
   skin cold to touch
   sad worried look

   b) self-concept mode

   identify with sisters problem
   can't concentrate asked time a lot.

   c) role function mode

   losing function as a complete women
   loss of income role being loss.

   d) interdependence mode

   reach out to nurse as friend being nice

2) List some nursing strategies to alleviate Mrs. V.'s anxiety and state your rationale.

   Review surgery   ask sister problems
   you appear worried? Would you like to talk?
   Reassure pt will
   be in recovery room

70

CONCEPT OF ANGER AND HOSTILITY

Anger is a disruptive emotion or a feeling state which may be experienced by an individual in response to a frustration, conflict of motives, injury, insults, threats, and heightened anxiety.

Anger, perhaps more than any other emotions, is readily elicited and has many different modes of expression. An individual may reflect stages of anger changing from quiet and unresponsive behavior or passivity to feelings of rage and aggression that may lead to violence either physical or verbal.

The essential condition for eliciting anger is the blocking of a desired goal, especially when there is repeated and persistent prevention of the goal attainment. At first the person may feel nothing more than a slight sense of exasperation or frustration, but with prolonged exposure to this type of situation, the individual may become quite angry and may even reach a state of rage or fury with the resultant increase in tension and corresponding physiological manifestations. Unfortunately situations where goal attainment is blocked are inevitable and so are the emotions these situations generate. Even as babies, he or she may experience situations in which gratification may be delayed, and the infant being toilet trained or taught to eat food properly with a spoon, will yield to the parental influence with concomitant frustration. In a complex, modern society where the good of many takes priority over the satisfaction of individual desires, people are constantly faced with situations where goal attainment must be delayed. There may be times when individuals feel that other people are always standing in their way preventing them from obtaining what they want. The teenager who is not allowed to go on a weekend trip with some friends may feel a great deal of anger towards the blocking agents, in this case, the parents.

Hostility, on the other hand, may be viewed as a continuum where the expression of which may range from overly polite behavior to the opposite end of the spectrum of being totally consumed by intense uncontrollable expression of behavior. According to various theorists, hostility is the tendency of a person to do something harmful to others and to oneself; aggression may have a constructive meaning and need not be hostile just as hostility may be passive and not aggressively expressed; nor can one equate hostility with anger which is usually short-lived while hostility is a feeling of chronic antagonism and resentment which is accompanied by a wish to hurt and humiliate others.

Covert expression of hostility may be frequent but not always identified. For example, an individual may become quiet because he is resentful or withdraws from a perceived threat while seething with anger for being unable to cope with the threat. Overt expression of hostility may take the form of sarcastic and fault-finding remarks, rejection, argumentative and demanding verbal attacks, or even hostile jokes.

In recognizing that anger occurs as a result of frustration and unfulfilled needs, it is generally agreed that there are two main sources of stressors that exist, namely:

a) environmental—those that are externally and socially imposed, ranging from poor weather when an outing is planned, to working for a very controlling boss who appears determined to make life miserable for an employee, the systematic condition aimed at suppressing or extinguishing angry responses and many more.
b) personal—certain other frustrations occur as a result of deficits within an individual which reduce or eliminate the chance of attaining certain objective. For example, a person with limited intellectual abilities aspiring to become a nurse may be screened out by the variety of hurdles that must be crossed merely to be accepted into nursing school.

Disease or physical impairment may also prove to be a source of frustration by preventing the individual from leading a chosen life style. Certain self-imposed restrictions in life style can also lead to frustration and, as a result, irritability. A number of other factors, including mood, physical well-being, situations, past experiences and view of the blocking agent, may lower frustration tolerance and increase the potential for an angry reaction.

Not all stressors will lead to anger. A great deal seems to depend upon the extent to which there is an identifiable barrier to goal achievement. If the person can understand or label what is preventing success, anger is not likely to occur, but if the person sees rightly or wrongly an obstacle that is causing the difficulty, particularly if unreasonable or malicious motives are ascribed to the individual, anger is more likely to occur and will be directed towards the identified object.

The expression of anger can lead to positive feelings of power and potency. This occurs when it is focused directly at the source of the frustration and expressed in a socially appropriate, constructive manner. Under these conditions, anger may lead to positive social change and the resultant improvement in the individual's self concept. If on the other hand anger is misdirected or expressed in a socially inappropriate manner, this will lead to alienation, further frustration and depletion of coping abilities and loss of control.

Essential Aspects of Anger or Hostility:
– it may be turned inward to oneself or it may be expressed directly or projected overtly toward others and the environment
– it may be experienced consciously or unconsciously
– ways of expressing anger vary and change with age, culture, life style and goals
– it can be a conditioned generalized response
– if dealt with constructively, it leads to positive change of self
– if misdirected or destructive, it leads to increased frustration, further alienation and low self-concept

Any illness is to some extent confining and frustrating which eventually leads to anger. The emotional tone in client's condition should be given some attention, and it is regrettable that these factors are often relegated to a secondary position. An effective and caring nurse will be ever mindful that anger may be hidden behind symptoms of numerous complaints. Similarly, nurses need to be aware of their own responses to angry feelings to be ready at all times to intervene on client's behalf.

ASSESSMENT
BEHAVIORAL MANIFESTATION OF ANGER

Physiological Mode	Self-Concept Mode	Role Function Mode	Interdependence
– increased salivation	– loss of control	– inability to function	– aggression
– nausea and vomiting	– low frustration level	– aggressive or nonassertive	– demanding
– increased respiration, pulse rate and blood pressure	– increased alertness although fragmented	– impaired judgement	– fault finding
– dilatation of pupils	– low self-esteem	– abusive behavior as identified from previous experiences	– argumentative
– increased muscle tension	– worthlessness		– easily provoked
– restlessness, agitation	– guilt		– temper tantrums
– increased or decreased gastric motility	– destructive coping with anger		– revengeful
– frequency of urination			– isolation
– increased or decreased hydrochloric secretions			– physical combativeness
			– uncooperative
			– negative attitude

PLANNING AND IMPLEMENTATION

Strategies	Rationale
Physiological Mode – observe fluid and nutritional intake, elimination and sleep patterns	– establish and maintain adequate nutrition, hydration, elimination and rest
– engage client in physical activities	– to re-direct the expression of anger constructively – to displace energy associated with anger into a more socially acceptable way
– decrease environmental stimuli	– to provide a non-stimulating environment as client is easily provoked and irritated
Self-Concept Mode – calmly stay with client	– to reassure client that nurse is present to control situation as client is usually fearful that he/she might get out of control again – to convey acceptance to client without fear of retaliation
– provide period of "settling down"	– to display respect and preserve integrity for the client – to provide opportunity for the client to regain composure
– assist client to express feelings of anger and hostility	– to help client identify and become aware of these feelings – to assess whether anger is turned inward or projected into environment – to decrease client's hostile behavior through ventilation – help client understand that his/her behavior is a result of anger
Role Function Mode – increase client's ability to control behavior as a result of anger	– to utilize energy into a more constructive way – to develop problem solving skills in coping with anger
– assist client to seek other ways of relating to others without need to resort to defensive behavior	– to improve relationship with others – to help client view behavior as loss of control
– do not use physical restraints as much as possible	– to allow certain freedom to move around within limits – to convey non-invasion of client's own space and territory – to prevent client from feeling trapped
Interdependence Mode – determine the need for PRN medication	– to provide for the safety needs of the client and others
– discuss with client his/her feelings toward others	– to improve relation – assist client understand how he/she relates to others
– identify sources of anger and hostility	– to help client locate sources of anger and hostility which may be related to past experiences and relation with others – separate client with those other clients who are mutually antagonistic

EVALUATION

– Evaluate effectiveness of nursing actions.
– Modify and propose alternative nursing actions.
– What factors influenced or hindered the effectiveness of your nursing actions?

ANGER I

Duration: 5 minutes

Direction: Complete the following statements

1. I got angry this week when _____

2. When I feel angry I behave like _____

3. After I behave that way I feel _____

4. Whenever I get angry I feel like _____

5. I know that I am angry when _____

6. The person involved in my anger was _____

7. When I get angry I want people to _____

8. I get angry when people _____

9. When people get angry I usually _____

10. To alleviate my feelings of anger I usually _____

_____

Exercise 20

ANGER II

Duration: 10 minutes

Direction: Read the situation and answer the questions.

You attended a dinner dance with your boyfriend. Upon arrival, you saw his ex-fiancee sitting with some of her friends. Your boyfriend excused himself and approached his former girlfriend and spent most of the evening with her.

1) Identify your reactions to the above situation according to:
   a. physiological mode

   b. self-concept mode

   c. role function mode

   d. interdependence mode

2) State possible reasons for your behavioral responses.

3) List the various coping behaviors that you have utilized according to:

Constructive Coping   *Destructive Coping*

Exercise 21
ANGER III

Duration: 10 minutes

Direction: State 10 statements or comments from a client that will reflect anger or hostility

1. _____

2. _____

3. _____

4. _____

5. _____

6. _____

7. _____

8. _____

9. _____

10. _____

CONCEPT OF LOSS

Loss, in its broadest sense, means relinquishing of a valued or significant object. It involves loss of function whether it be in part or in whole and it encompasses many facets ranging from simple loss of a significant object to a more complex loss associated with death and dying. It refers not only to body parts and their functions, but also to deprivation of personally significant needs and values such as loss of self-esteem, employment, significant others through separation or divorce, familiar environment, role, and so forth. The emotional responses to the loss, whether concrete or symbolic, will be greater if the person has been emotionally involved in the relationship or possession. The emotional responses will take the form of a grief reaction and manifest a unique behavioral response.

The psychological phenomena of loss are usually followed by "grief" which is often used to describe the suffering, sorrow and failure experienced by the individual. It is the emotional part of mourning.

Mourning is a social process that refers to the culturally patterned expression of the bereaved person's thoughts and feelings and the corresponding social behavior that deals with death reflecting the attitudes and customs of a given society. "Grieving" on the other hand, is the psychological process which is necessary to overcome the subjective state of grief that follows the loss.

"Anticipatory grief or preparatory grief" is the grief prior to any loss or death experienced by either the family or client or both. It is a way of beginning to adapt to an impending loss, keeping the emotional responses within certain bounds but not eliminating the impact of the actual loss or death. In an attempt to bring oneself into a state of homeostasis, a series of behavioral responses is generated as the person goes through the grief and grieving process.

The illustration that follows demonstrates the similarities in the stages and responses in grief and grieving process whether the loss is a reaction to a crisis, death or dying, either by the client or the family member.

It will also serve as a useful guide for nurses when it is time to act as well as to talk when he or she is to be with a dying client and the members of the family.

Many nurses have approached a dying client with trepidation, expecting a scene or demand that he or she cannot possibly cope with. It may well be that there is a need to become increasingly aware of one's own thoughts about life and death to be able to come to terms in dealing with dying clients. There is no proven way to be with a dying person except to relate to him or her with the best qualities that nurses are able to bring to similar nurse-client relationships. Being your own self can be the most effective and helpful way of being with a dying client because the nurse can then keep the client in contact with at least one authentic point of interpersonal relation rather than saying something that is carefully rehearsed.

Stages of Grief and Grieving	Psychological Stages of Dying	Emotional Reaction to Physical Trauma and Crises
1. *SHOCK AND DISBELIEF*—denial, stunned, numb feelings, intellectual response to loss, carry activities automatically, motionless	1. *DENIAL STATE*—"No, not me!"	1. *IMPACT*—initial encounter which leaves the individual in a state of psychological shock—depersonalization. Sensations and emotions are not distinguished; poorly controlled behaviour, numbness, feelings associated with other events.
2. *DEVELOPING AWARENESS OF THE LOSS*—acute increasing anguish, feeling of emptiness and loss, anger, crying to acknowledge loss, reinforce dependency to lost object.	2. *ANGER STATE*—"Why me?"—become demanding, difficult and angry at anything that represents life. Begins to worry about family, may start taking precautions.	2. *RETREAT*—although physiological responses are normal, psychological attempt to deny existence of change exist; becomes angry, fights back; reality perception is distorted, indifferent to crisis, denies pain or symptoms, unrealistic plans for the future.

Figure 5.1 Concept of Loss

Figure 5.1—*Continued*

Stages of Grief and Grieving	Psychological Stages of Dying	Emotional Reaction to Physical Trauma and Crises
3. *RESTITUTION*—start of mourning phase to initiate recovery process, rituals of funeral service to emphasize reality of death, sharing of grief with family and friends.	3. *STATE OF BARGAINING*—"Yes me, but . . .". Bargaining is usually with God. Initiation of acceptance.	3. *ACKNOWLEDGMENT*—stage where reality of loss must be accepted if recovery is to occur, goes into mourning period, search for new self-image, isolation, argumentative, sarcastic, anger due to rebellion and feeling of unworthiness.
4. *RESOLVING THE LOSS*—"grief work" continues intrapsychically. It involves a number of steps which proceed haltingly at intervals, namely: (a) attempts to deal with the pain of loss (b) cannot accept new object to replace loss but may accept passive dependent relationship with family (c) becomes more aware of own body and various bodily sensations which are identical with the deceased. (d) preoccupation with the deceased.	4. *ACCEPTANCE STATE*—"Yes, me." Acknowledges that his time has come. - becomes depressed - emotionally detached - weeps by himself, silent - prefers to be with loved ones ――――――― 5. *PREPARATORY GRIEF*	4. *RECONSTRUCTION*—stage where feelings appropriate to the loss is abandoned; mourning is replaced by a decision to try a new beginning. Utilizes sublimation and compensation. Regressive tendencies are expected from time to time until mastery of the loss is accomplished. As changes in behaviour occur, new experiences will emerge to strengthen the integration process and increase the motivation.
5. *IDEALIZATION*—all negative and hostile feelings towards the deceased are repressed. Two important changes occur, namely: (a) distinct image of the deceased is established which is devoid of undesirable traits. (b) identification of desirable qualities of the deceased.		

ASSESSMENT
BEHAVIORAL MANIFESTATION OF GRIEVING PROCESS

Physiological Mode	Self Concept Mode	Role Function Mode	Interdependence Mode
– loss of appetite – insomnia – tightness in the throat – choking with shortness of breath – lack of muscular power – poor concentration – poor memory – numbness – loss of weight – circulatory collapse	– denial – anger – guilt – withdrawal – powerlessness – reality perception may become distorted – somatic distress, i.e. empty abdominal feeling, pain, tension – neglect of self care	– high risk to self and others – careless on the job – cannot recognize potential hazards at work – cannot function as readily as usual – refusal to perform activities of daily living even though physically capable	– becomes overly dependent on family and others – regression – alienation from family and friends – withdrawn

Physiological Mode	Self Concept Mode	Role Function Mode	Interdependence Mode
– absence of corneal reflex – visible physical and mental deterioration	– preoccupation of the deceased and/or preoccupation of fear and dying – altered body image – depression – self destructive		

PLANNING AND IMPLEMENTATION

Strategies	Rationale
Physiological Mode – observe the fluid and nutritional intake, elimination, sleep and activity patterns	– to maintain eating habits, sleep and activity patterns which are impaired due to physiological responses of the grieving process – to prevent further loss of weight, maintain hydration and attain optimal level of health and functioning – to assist in coping with the physical stress brought about by the loss
– provide for physiological needs, i.e. personal hygiene, comfort measures	– to keep client as comfortable as possible – to maintain dignity and integrity of the client – to provide physical contact to allay apprehension of being alone and dying
– observe closely changes in physiological responses	– to determine evidence of imminent death
Self-Concept Mode – establish rapport	– to facilitate trust and promote consistency
– spend some time with client	– to discern pattern of grieving process – to provide physical contact especially if frightened – to discern client's desire to ventilate – to become aware when to withdraw so client can work through the grieving process – to facilitate a supportive environment
– assist client to express feelings about the loss	– to convey acceptance of feelings and means of expression as clients experiencing loss have a desire to discuss own feelings and thoughts – to facilitate progression of grieving process through the stages and convey to client that these feelings, although painful, are normal and necessary to complete the grief work – to decrease denial of the loss, guilt, anger toward the lost object, and facilitate acceptance
– identify sources of loss	– to provide realistic appraisal of loss. For example, perception of altered body image is more significant than the complete loss of disability

Strategies	Rationale
Role Function Mode – explore emotional and role changes as a result of the loss	– to provide opportunity to develop alternative responses and adapt to new role changes
– assist in future planning with regard to changes	– to become aware of the limitations due to loss
	– to facilitate realistic planning and setting of future goals
	– to maintain problem-solving skills
	– to encourage normal performance of daily activities of living in spite of the loss
Interdependence Mode – encourage to talk to other clients about the loss	– to discourage dependency on staff members
	– to facilitate sharing, communication, ventilation of feelings and gain support
	– to discuss own feelings about self, toward others and the lost object
– inform other staff members of client's reaction to the loss	– to determine the need for referral, i.e. psychiatric consultation, need for clergy, social work and so forth

EVALUATION

– Evaluate effectiveness of nursing actions.
– How did your own thoughts and feeling about death and dying influence or hinder your nursing approaches?
– What was the attitude of the family and other staff members toward the loss?

Exercise 22

LOSS

Duration: several hours prior to class

Direction: Role play the following situations for several hours.

- blindness: wear dark glasses and use a cane
- inability to walk: use crutches or a wheelchair
- deafness: place earplugs in your ears
- speech impediment: stutter or lisp
- immobility: stay in one position and pretend to be unable to walk
- loss of any significant body possessions

1. Identify your responses according to physiological, self-concept, role function and interdependence modes.

2. Note how others will react to you:

3. What support system did you find most helpful?

Exercise 23

DEATH AND DYING

Duration: 15 minutes

Direction: We know that many people have difficulties with the word "death". People react to the term with morbidity rather than reality. The critical question here is the far-reaching implication of one's attitude toward death and oneself, and how these attitudes influence the health workers' therapeutic stance to humanize and dignify the process of death.

To help you assess some of your personal views about death and you, please answer the choice which mostly applies to you.

1. As a child, how was the topic of death discussed in your family?
   1) never
   2) cautiously
   3) openly
   4) with discomfort

2. Have you ever experienced death in your family? If yes, did it affect your attitude toward your own death?
   1) yes
   2) no
   3) sometimes

3. How do you feel when you think of your own death?
   1) anxious
   2) sad
   3) relieved
   4) glad to be alive

4. Which of the following is most anxiety-provoking for you whenever you think of your own death?
   1) dying without your significant other
   2) dying away from home
   3) dying alone and suddenly
   4) the manner of dying

5. What aspect of death is most distasteful to you?
   1) uncertainty of life after death
   2) fear of body decomposition
   3) grief of the family
   4) process of dying

6. If given the choice, when would you like to die?
   1) adolescence age
   2) middle age
   3) after retirement
   4) old age

7. What does death mean to you?
   1) finality of life
   2) beginning of a new life
   3) meaningful cessation
   4) fulfillment of life's meaning and goals

8. If you had a choice, what manner of death would you prefer?
   1) sudden death
   2) violent death
   3) natural death
   4) do not care

9. If you are dying of terminal illness, would you prefer to be informed?
   1) yes
   2) no

10. If you were told that you were dying, how would you spend your time until the time of your death?
    1) I would change my life style
    2) I would not change my life style
    3) I would keep my estate in order
    4) I would prepare myself spiritually

11. What kind of funeral services would you prefer?
    1) memorial service only
    2) traditional services
    3) elaborate formal services
    4) informal services

12. Would you approve of an autopsy being performed on you?
    1) yes
    2) no
    3) it depends on the circumstances

13. How would you like to have your body disposed of?
    1) burial
    2) cremation
    3) donation
    4) do not care

14. What are your thoughts about leaving a will?
    1) I already have one
    2) I intend to make one
    3) I do not wish to leave one
    4) I am not sure

15. At present I have discussed with my family and friends
    1) all of the above thoughts and feelings
    2) some of the above thoughts and feelings
    3) none of the above
    4) I have not discussed any of the above

CONCEPT OF GUILT

The sense of guilt is a concept of great significance in psychology and psychiatry because it is the forerunner of most emotional problems and psychiatric symptoms. To gain better understanding of guilt it is helpful to consider the development of super ego and its functions since it is the expression of tension between the ego and the super ego.

The development of guilt is a gradual process and follows the appreciation of right and wrong which has been initiated in the early years of life. A child may accept the parents' dictum when told that a thing is good or bad but inner feelings, commonly known as conscience, are seldom apparent until the child begins to display definite feelings that may be called guilt when he or she has done something wrong, even though the child may not be found or reprimanded by the adults.

The conviction of wrong doing is often intensified by the intimidation and fear that one's upbringing instills into the immature and developing mind. It is impossible, therefore, for anyone wholly to escape guilt feelings.

The real harm that flows from past experiences is entirely mental and it produces so much unwarranted guilt that it eventually dominates the adult life. It may be said that one's guilt potential is then in direct proportion to one's social development.

Guilt is the root cause for fears of all kinds; for shame, oversensitiveness, discouragement and disgust, self-pity, conviction of unworthiness and failure, despair, morbid self-depreciation, uncertainty and vascillation and all types of mental tortures, not to mention the physical symptoms that it produces.

Although all people are more or less experiencing these feelings at some points of their lives, only when such feelings become pronounced and disproportionate, do they become symptoms of a more profound emotional conflict and psychiatric problems. It is perhaps worth noting that a well adapted conscience only evokes guilt when feelings are realistic and appropriate to the situation rather than evoking guilt in actions that elicit punitive responses that probably have no direct or significant relation to the present situation.

Guilt related to past experiences of the individual are generated not so much from what one has done as from what one has unconsciously wished to do.

It may be conscious to the perception that it has failed to perform the ideal when at variance with or contrary to the standard one has set for oneself.

In an unconscious level it may be perceived as need for punishment for past unacceptable behavior and/or for becoming a burden to others, for example, becoming ill, causing pain to others, misfortunes, and so forth.

Guilt like other feelings is often repressed for fear of retaliation and rejection. As a result, the individual may no longer be conscious of the guilt and lose touch with the feelings but the coping behaviors may become more obvious in an attempt to deal with the disagreeable emotions linked to guilt.

It is not uncommon for nurses to see a whole constellation of coping behaviors, both direct and indirect, that might be generated from such a psychological state. A client with overwhelming guilt may give up when stricken by a relatively minor ailment and allow his or her condition to worsen, or reduce his or her activities so drastically that both mind and body are in poor tone to respond to any kind of stress. Similarly, the burden-beyond-bearing guilt may have much to do with the development of psychiatric problems and such conditions suggest that guilt is a concept deserving careful and systematic attention that will contribute to a more sensitive care and understanding.

ASSESSMENT
BEHAVIORAL MANIFESTATION OF GUILT

Physiological Mode	Self-Concept Mode	Role Function Mode	Interdependence Mode
– see Anxiety section – scoriated skin due to extensive handwashing	– worthlessness – self-depreciation – distorted perception of rightness and wrongness – strict adherence to moral and ethical standards – displeasure with own behavior – punitive behaviors – depression – anxiety	– commonly subscribe to punitive role function – sets high expectation of performance on self and others – oversolicitousness – strict adherence to role function	– ritualistic activities – disatisfaction with achievement – inadequate problem solving skills – tend to isolate

PLANNING AND IMPLEMENTATION

Strategies	Rationale
Physiological Mode – see Anxiety section, Chapter V	– to establish and maintain nutrition as client may not eat due to guilt and may feel that he or she is unworthy of food
– observe for excoriated skin due to excessive handwashing	– food and fluid may be omitted as part of ritualistic behavior or preoccupation
– provide safety measures	– ritualistic behavior may develop in an attempt to eradicate guilt – to protect from harming self due to ritualistic behavior
Self-Concept Mode – encourage client to recall experiences that produce guilt	– to identify real sources of guilt – to discourage rumination
– assist client explore causes of guilt	– to provide opportunity to work through guilt feelings – to relate guilt with perceived causes
– help client anticipate ways to deal with guilt	– to facilitate growth in ability to express and deal with feelings of guilt – to explore and identify ways of relieving guilt
– avoid non-verbal approaches indicating disapproval	– to provide non-judgemental environment and attitude thus to decrease guilt
Role Function Mode – see Depression section	
– provide menial tasks	– to provide opportunity to relieve guilt as client commonly feels the need for punishment – to provide an outlet for tension brought on by guilt

Strategies	Rationale
– set clear expectation of performance	– to perform comfortably without evoking guilt
	– to reduce use of maladaptive behavior in performance if unable to achieve
– establish routine activities	– to avoid anxiety-provoking changes that may produce guilt if unable to perform
Interdependence Mode – assist in making decisions	– to reduce anxiety in problem-solving thus preventing or reducing ritualistic behavior
– assign simple tasks	– to provide opportunity in which positive accomplishment can be made

EVALUATION

– Evaluate effectiveness of nursing actions.
– Modify and propose alternative nursing approaches.

Exercise 24

GUILT

Duration: 10 minutes

Direction:

1. List five common comments or statements that a client may express to indicate guilt.

2. How might these responses influence your role as a nurse? As a person?

CONCEPT OF POWERLESSNESS

In an attempt to understand the concept of powerlessness, much has been said about anxiety, anger, loss and guilt and its inter-relation which is further accentuated by alienation of the individual.

The need for power is often involved with the need for status since one way of achieving status is to gain power over others. By and large, human beings are motivated to achieve some status, whether the motive may consist of simply being well thought of, to have recognition and respect from others, or the desire to attain the highest possible position in the community. The need for power, however, can exist and be expressed independently of status need. Each individual has a personal need for control and power, control over one's being and environment. Whenever external or internal factors force the person to relinquish that control, he or she may feel detached, alienated and experience an overwhelming feeling of powerlessness.

The loss of control implies loss of power, and may be manifested in the following categories:

a. psychological loss of control which focuses on the individual's psychological structure and functioning, i.e. self-concept, role function, and interdependence
b. physiological loss of control which focuses on physical illness and early attitude toward the sick role

Therefore, powerlessness may be described as a "perceived lack of personal and internal control of events". Since it is commonly associated with anxiety, anger, loss and guilt, the behavioral responses will not be discussed but the learner needs to refer to the preceding sections of this chapter based on the assessed behavioral manifestation.

CONCEPT OF LONELINESS

Loneliness is only one emotion among many that is interrelated with other mental health concepts. Its significance has gained increasing recognition in the past few years due to man's need for relatedness, changes in family unit system, changes in role expectation, cultural mobility and so forth. The effects of loneliness in the individual's life will depend to a large extent on its intensity, duration and frequency. It is often mixed with other emotions, thus one can become quite anxious and withdraw from any anxiety provoking situation and feel isolated and lonely; one can feel quite lonely and attempt to cover this up with anger and hostility; one may experience loss and separation from significant others, objects or situations and feel abandoned and lonely; or one may be separated from the source of security and become powerless and feel guilt for being in this state.

Sullivan discussed the roots of loneliness as a result of early childhood experiences in which remoteness, indifference, and emptiness were the principal themes that characterized the child's relationship with others. The arrest in the socializing process at home did not prepare the child for contacts with peers in the next stages of the development and consequently the future relationship became a real and anticipated source of humiliation, punishment and anxiety. The real or imagined threats supported by the fear or error deepens the sense of social isolation and the evolving need to be right, to be able, coupled with feelings of failure and isolation from others, all help to nourish the developing sense of loneliness.

Lonesomeness, aloneness and loneliness are words frequently used interchangeably but without precise definition. In order to approach the concept of loneliness from within a frame of reference, it is important to establish a definition that can be used as a basis for continuing discussion.

According to various literatures, the feeling of lonesomeness is an experience that occurs at various times of life and implies being without the company of others but recognizing a wish to be with others. It can occur even when a person is alone or it can also be felt despite proximity to others in a group. The person recognizes his or her desire to feel closer to someone and is able to state it as a feeling and take actions to relieve the feeling of lonesomeness.

Aloneness also implies being without others but it is usually a highly personal and singular experience as the individual may choose to be alone without being lonesome to accomplish a particular goal. Being alone offers an opportunity for working through a particular kind of problem without any distractions and it is possible to be alone without being lonely or lonesome when seclusion and protected isolation are recognized and chosen as desirable for accomplishing specific tasks. It may also be experienced without choice as for example when the person makes some decisions in which he or she is alone in that act that will affect future planning.

Loneliness, on the other hand, is not a choice and it is somewhat different from aloneness and lonesomeness in that the lonely person is not aware of the feeling as such, is not aware of the reason why he does what he does when experiencing loneliness. Peplau defines it "as an unnoticed inability to do anything while alone".

Quite often, loneliness is not felt but the individual usually experiences a feeling of despair, separateness from something that is desired or needed, feel abandoned, apprehensive about the future, and feeling of being unloved and cared for even in the presence of significant others.

These feelings are so intense and unbearable that automatic responses or actions are precipitated forcing others to make contact with the lonely person. These behaviors govern the person's actions and eventually become a pattern of living which may seem senseless to others.

Another perspective from which to view loneliness is to know the two types of loneliness and its positive and negative functions, namely:

a. Existential loneliness is a state where the person becomes fully aware of oneself as an isolated solitary being. These feelings are related to the present experiences of the person which may involve physical and psychological pain. For example, the threat of presence of illness may create feeling of existential loneliness as it involves separation from significant others and familiar environment where the person may become more acutely aware of human separateness.

b. Loneliness Anxiety is a state of loneliness where anxiety is operating predominantly. The anxiety is chronic and diffused, emphasizing a basic alienation among individuals and people in relation of man to society. This state of loneliness is more concerned with fear of aloneness in the environment and the future implication of being alone.

In the course of loneliness, however, the person will be able to look at oneself and his or her responses to loneliness. Development of self-awareness would involve many thoughts and feelings one has about oneself, meanings the person gives to these experiences and how one would react. Consequently, awareness and acceptance of this existence can promote understanding, development of creativity thus facilitating growth—learning how to cope with various reactions and developing alternate ways to fill life and make it more fulfilling.

Similarly, denial of the existence of loneliness will not facilitate growth due to lack of appraisal of one's capabilities and limitations which are important to the integration of one's own self concept thereby causing lack of expression that will further accentuate feelings of isolation.

The adaptive and maladaptive responses to loneliness may be covert or overt and since loneliness is so dreaded and painful, it is usually disguised and therefore dissociated. Instead, defenses against loneliness determine the person's behavior and the patterns of defenses become automatic. The clients frequently offer plausible explanations of what he or she is doing and does not recognize the purpose of behavior and the efforts of attempting to ward off the evolving sense of loneliness.

Hence, the general cues to the needs of lonely clients are made available in the generic roots of the problem. When nurses can understand how loneliness has evolved, they can anticipate what kind of nurse-client relationship would be desirable or the type of relationship that may be traumatic and avoided so that he or she can avoid acting in ways that might reinforce the problem. The process of identification with the client's loneliness will depend upon the nurses' acceptance of his or her own feeling of loneliness and methods of coping. The ability to sense what it is and what the client is feeling will enable the nurse to intervene effectively and participate in this emotionally charged situation without being overwhelmed by feelings of her or his own loneliness.

Since the defenses or coping behaviors of the client are manifested and closely related to anxiety, anger, loss, guilt, depression, powerlessness and helplessness, the focus of nursing interventions for loneliness will be found in the sections.

Suggested Readings

Burd, S. F., Marshall, M. A., *Some Clinical Approaches to Psychiatric Nursing.* New York. Macmillan and Co., 1963

Bowlby, J., *Separation Anxiety.* The International Journal of Psychoanalysis. March-June, 1960

Carlson, C., *Behavioral Concepts and Nursing Intervention.* Philadelphia. J. B. Lippincott, 1970

Cattell, R. B. & Scheir, I. N., *Theory and Research on Anxiety—Anxiety and Behavior.* New York. Academic Press. 1966

Clark, C. C., *Nursing Concepts and Processes.* Albany, New York. Delmars Publishers, A Division of Litton Educational Publishing Inc., 1977

Dunlap, L. C., *Mental Health Concepts Applied to Nursing.* New York. A Wiley Medical Publication, 1978

Freud, S., *The Problem of Anxiety.* New York. Norton Press, 1963

Haber, J. et al., *Comprehensive Psychiatric Nursing.* 2nd ed., New York. McGraw-Hill Book Co., A Blakiston Publisher, 1982

Kreigh, H. Z. & Perko, J. R., *Psychiatric and Mental Health Nursing—Commitment to Care and Concern,* 2nd ed. Reston, Virginia. Reston Publishing Co., Prentice-Hall Co., 1983

Kyes, J. & Hofling, C., *Basic Psychiatric Concepts in Nursing,* 4th ed., Philadelphia. J. B. Lippincott, 1980

Noonan, K. A., *Emotional Adjustment to Illness.* New York. Delmar Publishers. 1975

Peplau, H. E., *Working Definition of Anxiety in Some Clinical Approaches to Psychiatric Nursing.* New York. MacMillan. 1963

Roberts, S., *Behavioral Concepts and Nursing Throughout the Life Span.* Englewood Cliffs, New Jersey. Prentice Hall, Inc., 1978

Roy, Sister C., et. al., *Introduction to Nursing: An Adaptation Model.* New Jersey. Prentice Hall, 1976

Spitz, R., *The Psychoanalytic Study of the Child.* New York. International University Press, 1965

CHAPTER 6

Protect eap

Defense Mechanisms

Defense mechanisms or mental dynamisms are mental devices utilized to a certain extent by everyone as a means of coping, relieving inner tensions or in resolving emotional conflicts. Although some mechanisms represent higher levels of adjustment in others, all will play some role in each person's life at some time. Since individuals differ greatly in their responses to life stresses and conflicts, these defense mechanisms may be classified either as adaptive or maladapative.

Adaptive responses involve modes of adjustment that represent fairly direct ways of dealing with problems. They are attempts to modify or change the situation while maladaptive responses involve excessive reliance on any one mechanism that results in pronounced degree of inappropriate utilization and may become prominent symptoms. Maladaptive defense mechanisms involve distortion of reality which is aimed at defending oneself against anxiety, are not directed toward changing the problems or conflicts and are commonly displayed by emotionally disturbed and mentally disturbed clients.

The following list describes the most common defense mechanisms.

Defense Mechanisms

Projection blaming others for one's own limitations, impulses and behavior. Projection occurs when we attribute our own thoughts and impulses to others. It is one method of removing our own conflicts and denying our limitations.

Displacement the discharge of emotions on safer sources rather than attacking the primary cause of the feelings. We may choose a substitute and release our feelings against him or her thereby displacing our feelings from the original anxiety-producing goal to another less threatening one.

Identification release of anxiety through identifying one's self with more powerful or prestigious persons or situations. It is also a means of acquiring social behavior by imitation of the persons we want to be like. Although similar with introjection, in introjection the process is more extensive and involves the assuming of values, beliefs and attitudes of other persons as a means of giving in to their wishes.

Compensation the concealing of felt or real inadequacies through emphasizing areas that provide reward or gratification. It is stressing or overemphasizing areas of skill or proficiency to offset areas in which we feel inadequate or frustrated. It can be a desirable and useful mechanism as compensatory behaviors direct attention away from limitation and develop skills in a non-handicapped area.

In overcompensation, however, this is carried to such an extreme that the person becomes inflexible and poorly adjusted as he has little to offer other than his area of overcompensation.

Substitution the replacement of a desired but frustrated goal by a less socially desirable expression. Although similar with sublimation, the frustrated motive in substitution is replaced by a behavior which is socially disapproved.

Sublimation the replacement of a forbidden or guilt producing activity with a socially acceptable behavior.

Rationalization	justification of one's behavior in a rational or reasonable manner providing a "good" excuse for one's actions. It allows us to meet our needs and provides an explanation for the behavior which is socially acceptable, rather than the real reasons, and are ones that one can live with more comfortably.
Suppression	making a conscious decision not to act.
Repression	the blocking out or denial of painful or dangerous thoughts from conscious awareness. It is the selective forgetting we do as a way of relieving ourselves of painful or distressing thoughts.
Regression	retreat to a previous less mature level of adjustment. Although similar with fixation, the regressed person has shown a higher or more mature level of adjustment, but due to traumatic experiences in meeting his needs, he has regressed to earlier periods in which frustrations were less and needs more easily met.
Fixation	arresting of emotional adjustment on an immature level through frustration of attempts at a higher level of adjustment. It differs from regression in that the fixated individual has never progressed beyond his primitive level of adjustment.
Reaction Formation	the denial of threatening though desired emotions and developing an attitude or action which is directly opposite to the actual wish.
Denial	acting as if the present or past situation is not happening or has not happened.
Intellectualization	utilization of technical terms when asked for feelings responses.
Depersonalization	feelings of unreality about one's own body and loss of identity.
Conversion	the act of transforming feelings into physical symptoms.

Suggested Readings

Kolb, L. C., *Noyes' Modern Clinical Psychiatry*. 10th ed. Philadelphia. W. B. Saunders Co., 1982
Kyes, J. and Hofling, C. *Basic Psychiatric Concepts in Nursing*. 4th ed. Philadelphia. J. B. Lipponcott, 1980.
*Any Psychology textbooks or Psychiatric nursing textbooks.

Exercise 25
DEFENSE MECHANISMS I

adaptive

Duration: 10 minutes

Direction: Read carefully. Name at least 10 defense mechanisms in this situation. Identify the defense mechanisms by underlying the behavior that describes the defenses utilized. Write the defense mechanisms below and define.

Situation #1:

A. B., a 19 year old female student of plain appearance, who appears somewhat quiet and inhibited, has no intention of attending a skiing weekend in a club unless the guy in whom she has an interest asks her to. For a long time, A. B. has tried to impress this guy subtly by behaving like the other girls who have previously caught his eye, but to no avail, as she obviously lacks the social skills and stamina that the other girls have. Because of this social inhibition, A. B. often resorts to her artistic abilities of painting and music. However, to her surprise, the guy asked A. B. to go skiing for the weekend. A. B. is thrilled and looks forward to the event with overwhelming enthusiasm.

On Friday afternoon, a phone call came and her date informed her of the change of plans and apologized. She answered him quite nicely and told him that she herself is not really sure whether she should go or not. After he hung up the telephone, A. B. banged the receiver, slammed the door and cried in her room. After a while, she developed a headache, refused to eat supper or talk to any of her family. Late in the evening, she decided to go out for a short walk, and upon her return, A. B. told her mother how marvelous the walk was and that she preferred to have done that.

A. B. convinced herself that skiing is not her interest and it would have been a total loss if she went with this guy. Furthermore, the guy is a "turkey" anyway, so she says.

What defense mechanisms were utilized? State and define.

1. Identification — act girls

2. Sublim. — painting

3. Conversion — headache

4. Displacement — slam door

5. Denial — wanted to go

6. rationalization — no go anyway

Project — turkey

Regression - not aware of social inadequacies

95

7.

8.

9.

10.

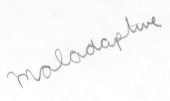
maladaptive

Exercise 26

DEFENSE MECHANISMS II

Duration: 10 minutes

Situation #2

During your interaction with your client, Mr. M. stated, "You nurses are all alike, and you always think that I refuse to participate in any activities . . . you are always after me." Then the client would go to one corner of the hall and would laugh and giggle to himself. While talking to him, you are told by Mr. M. that he misses his father and would like to go home and be with him . . . "On second thought, perhaps it would be better for me to stay here." When the Head Nurse called him saying, "Mr. M., you have a phone call", he refused to answer and stated that he is not Mr. M., "I am Little Jesus". Then he turned to you and stated "I am not really me. I am God". Oftentimes, Mr. M. really believes that he is God and says that people are crucifying him.

On occasion, Mr. M. talks to you rationally and when asked about his family, he firmly states that he does not remember. At times, he hits the wall with his fist when confronted if he does not participate in any given activities, giving reasons that he is in the hospital for his swollen leg.

What defense mechanisms were utilized by Mr. M.? List at least eight (8) defense mechanisms.

1. Projection

2. Denial

3. Displacement

4. Repression

5. identification

6. rationalization

7.

8.

Compare and contrast the use of above mechanisms with the defense mechanisms stated from Situation #1.

DEFENSE MECHANISMS III

Duration: 10 minutes

Direction: Match the correct definition with each of the mental mechanisms listed below.

1. Substitution
2. Compensation
3. Displacement
4. Sublimation
5. Repression
6. Reaction Formation
7. Denial
8. Suppression
9. Projection
10. Rationalization

_____ A. Conflict between two opposing emotions is avoided by keeping them apart in consciousness.

_____ B. Explaining one's emotions in an acceptable way while overlooking unacceptable emotions.

_____ C. An emotion is transferred from its actual object to a substitute.

_____ D. Refusal to acknowledge the existence of an emotion.

_____ E. Energy which is not socially acceptable in one situation is channeled into another situation where its expression is acceptable.

_____ F. A deliberate and conscious postponement of dealing with an emotion.

_____ G. An attempt to disguise an undesirable trait by emphasizing a desirable one.

_____ H. Accepting an object in the place of another desired object that one was unable to obtain.

_____ I. An attempt to control an undesirable drive by over-emphasizing the opposite one.

_____ J. A return to an earlier level of development.

_____ K. Attribute one's own emotions to another person.

_____ L. An emotion is excluded from conscious awareness and kept in the unconscious.

CHAPTER 7

The Depressed Client

How many people, both inside the hospital and out, suffer from depression? Depression is a problem that concerns everyone. So many people suffer from depression that none of us can escape some personal contact with them, and it is safe to say that everyone becomes depressed at some point in his or her life. The depression that we may experience, however, may not be so despairing as to attempt suicide but it is still an unpleasant experience that an individual goes through at some time or another. Depression is not only universal, but it also affects human beings irrespective of their gender, lifestyle, mentality, education, religion, and position in life. There are a great number of people who do not concede that they are experiencing depression for many fear that depression is acknowledging that they have some form of mental illness. Likewise, part of the problem of understanding depressive reactions is that the word "depression" has been used to describe such a wide variety of human psychological responses. When we say that everyone experiences depression, we are generally speaking of the many forms it takes. For example, the loss of a loved object, reaction to a particular situation, or even the change in weather. The natural struggle to meet one's needs will automatically cause emotional shifting, which will produce changes in behavior and in some instances, changes in appearance and activities.

Is depression normal? One point of view holds that all depression accurately defined is pathological and what has been commonly called depression is really sadness, sorrow or the blues. Hence the difference between normal and pathological depression will depend upon the severity of the symptoms, causative factors and ability of the individual to cope with the situation.

TYPES OF DEPRESSION

The tremendous increase in the number of depression today justifies a continuum behavioral approach to the types of depression varying from a mild degree or feeling state; moderate degree to mood disorder, and severe degree to a specific clinical syndrome. In a mild degree of depression, sometimes referred to as a "feeling state", the depression may manifest itself in the transitory feelings of sadness, disappointment, unhappiness and frustrations that are normal mood responses to any meaningful loss. In the more intense and prolonged depression, it can further occur along the continuum with devastating effect on the overall functioning of the individual and development of maladaptive responses.

Depression as a Feeling State	Depression as a Clinical Syndrome
- transient period of sadness brought on by disappointment or failures	- pathological state of dejection, despair, gloom
- tendency to weepiness	- crying spells accentuated
- aware of precipitating events	- total indifference
- lack of interest to pursue usual activities, but is able to function	- no insight; poor judgement
- lack of concentration	- total loss of interest and unable to function
- irritability, annoyance	- difficulty in concentration; slowed thinking process
- feelings of hopelessness	- detached, numbness
- feelings are self-limiting and normal sense of well-being is restored after a short period	- extreme feelings of helplessness and worthlessness
	- psychomotor retardation or agitation
	- extends for longer period; more stressful
	- characterized by specific criteria; affective disorder
	- suicidal ideation

Figure 7.1 States of Depression

Most psychiatric literature and textbooks recognize various types of depression in great detail according to its causation, intensity, duration and clinical manifestation. A more widely accepted view held by some authorities categorizes depression into: Depression as a feeling state and Depression as a clinical syndrome. For further study of the clinical types of depression, refer to Appendix A for DSM III classification.

THEORIES OF DEPRESSION

Although one may seek to understand depression in either psychosocial, biochemical and cognitive terms, these approaches are complementary. While depression generally begins in response to some real life situation or event, the depressive feelings pervade and may continue long afterwards and may develop into a more profound disturbance.

A. Psychodynamic Theories

Psychodynamic theories emphasize unconscious feelings and reactions in depressive reactions. According to psychodynamic approach, depression is a reaction to events that symbolize a bereavement. Freud and other theorists have emphasized the loss of a loved object and the loss results in the depletion of self which eventually leads to a reaction of mourning or grieving. The other most widely accepted explanation of the theory of depression from psychoanalytic framework is the classical Freudian view that depression is the result of a turning inwards upon the self of the anger, hostility and aggressive impulses which are previously directed outward. As a result, the individual perceives himself or herself as a worthless being who does not deserve any gratification.

Other professionals in the field focus on the history of disturbed early childhood relationship between the individual and his or her significant other, especially the mother figure. Some researchers and clinicians have reached the conclusion that severe depression may be rooted in rejection in early childhood. Other theorists discuss the significance of hostility, narcissistic needs and precarious self esteem. Others view depression as the discrepancy between the image of an ideal self and the real self. Accordingly, the ideal self is so perfect that the real self has difficulty attaining any qualities of the ideal self and in the process of self-actualization the distance between the two will make the individual threatened and resort to depression.

Somatic complaints and hypochondriasis of depressed persons may also represent narcissistic concerns with his own body image and by doing so the person may gain secondary and symbolic gain from self centering of attention and interest.

B. Cognitive and Learning Theories

The first theory proposed views the roots of depression as a negative mental set. It supposes that depression is the outgrowth of an insidious development of a negative self concept which generates to a negative view of the world, future and self. The label "optimist" and "pessimist" reflect the types of thinking that leads to depression. The depressed affective state is secondary to or caused by the negative cognitions.

Depressive episodes may be externally precipitated but it is the individual's perception and appraisal of the events that render it depression-inducing. Depressing thoughts and beliefs, false or accurate, lead to self deprecating statements which in turn lead to depression. Studies have shown that depressed individuals tend to focus more on negative or unpleasant material and literally screen out positive input. This is one of the reasons that depression seems to be self-perpetuating.

Other theories of depression are based on laboratory experiments with animals. Animals, given an experience in which they cannot escape or avoid unpleasant stimulus, behave passively when placed in new aversive context. This persists even in a new situation that would permit escape from the painful event. The previous experience with uncontrollable painful stimulus is believed to result in a form of "learned helplessness", which is characterized by a lack of motivation and inability to learn effective coping skills in new situations. In humans, this theory views reactive depression as a learned helplessness characterized most notably by the feeling of loss of control.

According to this model, if the person has experienced unpleasant events where there was no control over outcome, passive acceptance of a similar situation will be exhibited. This occurs even though a viable alternative is available. There is empirical support for this theory in the fact that the people who are experiencing depression usually feel that they have little control over significant events and appear to have given up.

The third theory is based on instrumental learning in that individuals are primarily motivated by reward and punishment. This theory states depression is due to an individual's low rate of response which is contingent to positive reinforcement. Three basic explanations are offered for the existence of the low rate of reinforcement, mainly, few events are reinforcing for the person; few reinforcing events are available in the particular environment; or the individual, perhaps due to lack of skills, does not produce many responses that are likely to be rewarded.

C. Biochemical Theories

The clinical observations and current research have led to an increasing focus on the role of biochemical factors in depression. The biochemistry of depression has attracted increasing interest in recent years and it is now established that most severe depressions are accompanied by elevated serum cortisol, high abnormally intracellular sodium levels which usually reverts to normal when depression lifts. There is also evidence of depletion of catecholamine concentrations (epinephrine and norephinephrine) in the hypothalamus and brain stem which may be directly or indirectly responsible for mood changes. Conversely, excessive norepinephrine at certain receptor sites is responsible for the mania. Many authorities also attribute a sizeable number of depressions to biological or glandular malfunctions. Because some depressed people have responded to medications it is assumed that their problem was due to abnormal body function. Certain biological factors that are frequently considered are neurophysiological changes and endocrine abnormalities.

D. Genetic Theories

Some investigators in the field indicate that a single dominant autosomal gene showing incomplete penetrance is an essential prerequisite to the development of endogenous depression. Researchers who have studied people with bipolar disorders revealed a family history of similar conditions. Thus, there seems to be a major genetic component for bipolar disorders and there is much less evidence for genetic cause in unipolar depression.

Depression in Childhood and Adolescence

The normal-abnormal distinction is somewhat fuzzy when applied to the category of depressive states of childhood and adolescence. Initially, adults perceive the child's life as a decade of happiness, enjoyment, play and no responsibilities that the notion of depression is unthinkable. The behavior that may indicate depression is not perceived as predictors of depression but rather referred to as problem behavior associated with aggression.

Children and adolescents, like the adults, vary in their readiness to experience discouragement and in coping with stressful situations. If unhappiness occurs in childhood it is usually situational and transitory in nature unless, of course, the child comes from a broken home where instead of enjoying the security of his or her parents, the child is subjected to separation, anxiety and then probably depression. Similarly, illness and hospitalization which necessitates separation from the home situation may also evoke the feelings of depression. The threat of the loss of a loved object is a constant factor found in these negative moods. Some children show more profound degrees of withdrawal and depression in response to the loss and threats. Hospitalized infants, deprived of adequate maternal love show a syndrome called "anaclitic depression" which is manifested by a display of apathy, failure to thrive, developmental retardation, irritability, fatigue and exhaustion.

School age children and adolescents may show lability of mood, sadness, feelings of boredom, irritability, feelings of helplessness, rejection, unloved and hopelessness. In many instances, loss of appetite and weight, insomnia or somnolence may be quite evident. Inability to concentrate in school which results in failing grades, lack of social and peer interest, dissatisfaction, indecisiveness and negative self esteem are quite common. It is not uncommon that these behaviors are at times masked and are displayed in aggressive tendencies.

The above behavioral manifestation if seen in adults will indicate depression but if seen in children their significance and interpretation are less clear and is not usually termed as depression. Many authorities agree that the diagnosis of depression should not be established in children if possible. This point of view suggests that the problems displayed by children are not really symptomatic of depression but rather as part of growth and development and that such behaviors may be a normal reaction to the stress of growth, development, school and social adjustment.

Clinicians agree that if the above behaviors occur more frequently and do not dissipate with time as the process of growth and development proceeds, a diagnosis of depression may be justified.

Depression in the Elderly

An increasing problem with depression in the elderly deals primarily with adaptation to retirement, new relations, decreased mobility, financial decline, role conflict, the loss of significant other, and presence of other physical or medical conditions. Because of the influence of our society regarding the retirement age many people are retiring even though the elderly may still be as productive and as active. Everyone is familiar with the successful businessman who lived a very productive life but died a few years later without any real physical ailment after his retirement. In most cases the problem stems from lack of goals and interest when one reaches this age. Consequently, the person becomes not only depression prone but also a morality risk. It appears that depression-free living is determined by one's contribution to the well being of others, the ability to adapt to the loss by replacement of such losses through new interests, associations, new roles, retraining of loss capabilities and to relatively keep active to retain healthy physical and mental functioning.

Preoccupation with self during the period of later years is a natural and dangerous threat to one's own well being. It is not uncommon to find the elderly engaging in self-pity, withdraw into their own selves and live in the past. Decrease of functions in this age period through disuse can also lead to unnecessary physical limitations, social alienation, disorientation, apathy and depression.

Surprisingly enough, the ninth decade of life does not seem to be more infused with depression. Some suggest that this is because people return to a child-like behavior and attitude towards life at this age. Others state that some individuals have already brought on a premature death and thus are more optimistic in their outlook on life.

The clinical picture of depression in the elderly resembles the behavioral manifestation found in the younger age group. Guilt and gross retardation are less common, but hypochondriasis, agitation, obsession and preoccupation with poverty are more pronounced. Projections and denial are the common defense mechanisms utilized in this age group.

Physical symptoms are more prominent and in fact it may be the first manifestation of depressive conditions. Weepiness may also be often exhibited although at times they may not be able to cry but feel like crying. Such clients give complaints of physical pain especially backaches, headaches or shoulder pains of long standing nature but they deny the feelings of depression. Occasionally, they may state feelings of hopelessness in relation to the physical complaints. Depression in this age group can vary greatly in intensity, duration and degree. Many elderly may just experience fleeting episodes of sadness, fatigue, temporary loss of interest and somatic complaints and often in response to an obvious loss. Others may experience a more pronounced, severe and long lasting depression without any obvious identifiable cause.

Interestingly enough, although one may not always be aware of it, there are similarities in the depression of an adolescent and the elderly in spite of the great differences in their ages. Both groups are intensely self-absorbed, often exhibit hypochondriasis, preoccupation with "nothingness" and death, pessimistic views about the future and often suffer from role conflict and adjustment process. In retrospect, each stage of growth and development of life offers its own potential cause of depression.

SUICIDE

The severity of depression together with the risk factors described in the Table of Risk Factors for Potential Suicide may cause the individual to become suicidal.

In almost every case of suicide the person experiences feelings of ambivalence, that is, the desire to live and at the same time the desire to die. Consequently, the person gives clues of the struggle against suicidal intent, the general message being a cry for help which may take the form of either direct or indirect verbal cues and behavioral communications.

Although suicide and suicidal attempts are high and commonly associated with depression, suicide varies from person to person, country to country and from one generation to the other. One cannot ignore the role of cultural differences, beliefs and values of the individual. Although suicide is a highly personal act there is also a profound social, philosophical and moral impact. In Japan, for example, the act of "hara-kiri" is considered an honourable action; "suttee" is a practice of culturally sanctioned suicide in India when the Hindu widow requests to be burned on her husband's funeral pyre to prove she has been a true and faithful wife; the Eskimos commit suicide when they are old and become a burden on the community; whereas in other countries, suicide is considered a cowardly act.

Dynamics of Suicide

From psychological point of view, suicide is motivated by feelings of hopelessness and worthlessness, a wish for revenge, and fantasies of being reunited with the lost object. The person rationalizes after progressively failing to cope with or adapt to multiple personal and environmental difficulties that the situation and distress are intolerable and seemingly unresolvable. At this point, the person feels helpless, useless, worthless and unwanted. These feelings of pessimism, hopelessness, unloved and having no one to live for are probably responsible for high suicide rates of the elderly, for those who are in physical pain, for those living alone, for widows without any children, and for the unmarried. Suicide attempts among the young often represent an expression of hostility towards someone or as an attempt to bring someone to terms. These motives are rare in the elderly as the older age group almost always fully intend to die. Suicidal preoccupation may also revolve not only around one's own feelings and failures but may be directed to other people's failure or aggressions which are directed towards himself or herself. The person may then begin to fantasize using suicidal acts or threats of it to resolve the problem by maneuvering other people into changing their attitudes and mainly to evoke feelings of guilt.

From sociological theories of suicide the key factor is social isolation, societal anxieties and lack of support system. Starting with the process of social development in infancy the person becomes interdependent in a social system, modes of behavior and personality traits are molded in part by mutual interchange of reinforcement and through interaction, the person's need for contact, belonging, affiliation, approval, status and power are satisfied. When the notion of social system is disrupted, relations and affiliations are discontinued and the individual reacts strongly against anyone who threatens his or her existence and these may be directed towards one's own self. The individual then becomes extremely lonely, isolated, fearful, pessimistic and helpless in forming meaningful relations which leads to alienation. These factors in turn may provide some clues to personal predisposition and may lead a person to attempt suicide.

Suicide can also occur in most mental disorders although the motives of such an act may be different. On the average, one third of the people who commit suicide have been suffering from neurosis, psychosis or severe personality disorders. It is rare among the mentally retarded, organic brain syndrome and the manic state in which the main symptom is elation with an exaggerated feeling of well being.

As previously stated, other dimensions to be considered in the overall causation of suicide is the cultural factors and incentives of the person. Family structure, occupational and achievement demands, responsibilities and economic condition are also significant aspects that need to be incorporated in assessing the crisis state of suicide.

In sum, the following Table outlines the risk factors for potential suicide that will be useful in the nursing assessment process.

Factors	High Risk	Low Risk
- Gender	- Male, More Successful	- Female, higher percentage of suicidal attempts
- Age	- Male-50 years & up - Female-25-50	- Under 25 years, although on the increase among the young and college students
- Race	- Caucasians - Orientals - Black-under 50	- Black-over 50
- Marital Status	- Divorced, separated - Widowed, single	- Married
- Religion	- No religious affiliation	- Strong religious ties
- Social Factors	- Professionals - Upper class - Urban areas with much social disorganization, isolation, alienation	- Middle and Lower class - Rural areas - Close family structure
- History of suicide	- Personal or family	- History of threats
- Lifestyle & Behavioural pattern	- Drinking and drug abuse - Acting out and impulsive behaviours - Emotional instability - Unstable pattern at work and no family ties	- Stabilized pattern of family life and work
- Precipitating Events	- Loss, actual or potential i.e.: death, illness, job, separation - Presence of other intolerable, numerous stressors	- Coping effectively with stress or crisis
- Time	- When depression is lifting - Early morning hours - Early summer, winter - Anniversaries, birthdays, suicide dates of famous people	- In depressive phase Autumn, except for a minor peak reported by some authorities
- Suicide Plan	- Premeditated, practice run - Specific plan - Availability of agents	- No definite plans
- Evidence of Maladaptive responses	- Agitated depression - Guilt feelings, self-deprecation, self-accusations, hopelessness, worthlessness, preoccupation with death - Fear of losing control, hurting others and self - Severe pain, somatic complaints - Insomnia, restlessness - Isolation from others - Direct or indirect communication of intent, i.e.: - "I am going to kill myself." - "I want to die." - "I will be better off dead." - "I cannot take this any longer." - "Goodbye, you will not see me anymore." - "I will not be here to be a burden to you." - "There's nothing left for me."	

Figure 7.2 Risk Factors for Potential Suicide

Figure 7.2—*Continued*

Factors	High Risk	Low Risk
	- Collection and hoarding of lethal agents - Getting affairs in order - Presence of other psychotic conditions - Ineffective coping skills	

ASSESSMENT
MALADAPTIVE RESPONSES TO DEPRESSION

I Physiological Mode	Mild Degree	Moderate Degree	Severe Degree
Alteration in: 1. Nutrition	– lack of interest in food – no appetite	– anorexia – omit meals without awareness – loss of weight	– anorexia – aversion to food – severe loss of weight – malnutrition
2. Sleep Pattern	– somatic complaints – restlessness during sleep – early awakening hours	– insomnia – sleeps most of the time – increase in restlessness and early awakening hours	– insomnia of longer duration – fretful and restless sleep – stupor
3. Optimal Activity	– tires easily – slow performance – reduction in physical activities – somatic complaints, backaches, headaches, stiff neck	– increased fatigue-ability – tiredness upon awakening – reduced performance – slow gait – lack of energy	– retarded performance or inability to perform – immobility – obvious evidence of lack of energy
4. Digestive Function	– altered elimination habits	– constipation or diarrhea – bad breath – preoccupation with gastrointestinal disturbances	– constipation – coating of tongue – bad breath
5. Sexual Activity	– lack of interest – reduced sexual responses	– marked reduction in sexual responses – loss of libido	– aversion to sex – unresponsive – amenorrhea
6. Thinking Process	– forgetfulness – some difficulty in concentration	– difficulty in concentration – slowed thinking, comprehension and verbal responses – somatic thought content; derogatory and suicidal intent	– retarded thinking process – decreased verbalization – mutism – persecutory and derogatory thought content – preoccupation with death; suicidal ideation – poverty of ideas

II Self Concept Mode	Mild Degree	Moderate Degree	Severe Degree
Alteration in: 1. Physical Self	– lack of social interest – neglect of self-care and grooming	– loss of interest in others – disinclination for usual pursuits – poor personal hygiene – distorted body image – change in body posture – self preoccupation – guilt and shame – self-accusatory	– indifferent to environment – unkempt, dishevelled appearance – immobile, detached – feels ugly, distorted repulsive – decreased muscle tone – stooped posture, furrowed brow, drooping and expressionless face
2. Moral Self	– shame and guilt – feeling of loss – disappointment, failure	– shame and guilt – self-accusatory	– guilt and remorse – suicidal ideation

III Role Function Mode	Mild Degree	Moderate Degree	Severe Degree
	– indecisiveness – feelings of inadequacy – diminished problem solving skills	– feelings of gloom and pessimism to foreboding feelings of helplessness, worthlessness and emptiness – shame and guilt	– feelings of gloom and pessimism to feelings of helplessness, worthlessness and emptiness – feelings of impending doom – powerlessness and loss – suicide as escape

IV Interdependence Mode	Mild Degree	Moderate Degree	Severe Degree
	– fear of rejection – social isolation – oversensitivity to others – dependent on others – non-participating	– extreme dependency and inadequacy – no motivation in performance – avoidance, escapist – seclusive – hostility – destructive to self/ others	– denial – complete withdrawal – seclusive – alienation – suicide as punishment

PLANNING AND IMPLEMENTATION

Strategies	Rationale
Physiological Mode – Assist with physical care appearance	– to promote personal hygiene. – to foster positive body image.
– Assist with nutrition	– to encourage client to eat. Client usually refuses meals, feels not worthy of food, is preoccupied – decreased activities dull the appetite – to prevent weight loss, emaciation and elimination problems
– Provide measures to induce rest and sleep	– to restore regular sleep patterns. Client may be restless, tense and agitated – disturbed sleeping signs are common, i.e.: frequent awakening, early awakening hours, insomnia – reduced physical activities, general physical condition, drugs and affective state reduce coping responses to stress and deplete physical and mental functions – unpredictable changes in bedroom routine preparations may augment sleep disturbances
– Provide physical activities	– to improve circulation, nutrition, elimination, muscle tone and body posture. Decreased activity impairs bodily functions – channel tension and agitations into constructive activity – to stimulate mental processes – to divert attention from self – to discourage preoccupation with morbid ideas and somatic complaints – to promote interaction with others
– Use simple statements during communication	– to allay feelings of inadequacy due to miscomprehension of statements. Client has difficulty in concentration, diminished ability to think that verbal responses may be slow and with great effort – interpretation of events may become distorted due to derogatory and persecutory nature of thought content

Strategies	Rationale
Self-Concept Mode – Spend time with client	– to demonstrate interest, concern and acceptance. Client feels worthless, unloved, rejected
	– to provide supportive measures against morbid impulses and self-punishment
	– to prevent increased seclusion and withdrawal
	– to provide safety in case of self-destruction especially when depression is lifting
	– attitude of hopefulness from staff conveys reassurance
	– to assist handling distressful feelings of depression
– Assist to verbalize feelings	– psychomotor retardation is present. Client has difficulty verbalizing, mental processes are slow
	– allow expression of verbal threats of suicide, subjective experiences, anger, guilt, hopelessness and worthlessness
	– explore sources of thoughts and feelings according to client's perception; relate distress to presence of feelings if client is ready
	– assist client to work through these feelings
	– discuss alternative methods of expression
	– externalization of feelings reduces aggression and sense of desperation
	– to assess further verbal and non-verbal clues of suicide, degree of ambivalence
	– to facilitate change of self-concept through discussion of personal strength
	– explore other options of coping methods
– Provide safety measures for suicidal client	– suicidal risk increases as depression begins to lift and motor retardation decreases
	– attempted threats are danger signs of potential suicide; do not ignore threats
	– to reduce environmental hazards such as checking belongings with client for lethal agents after thoughtful explanations; hoarding of sharp instruments, weapons, drugs; restriction on client's mobility
	– to convey interest and concern for the safety and feeling of security of the client
	– determine if possible the intensity and motive of suicide. Suicide may be an act of revenge, absolution from guilt or attempt to control others
	– determine the risk factors involved
	– allow expression of suicidal threats; do not argue with threats; suicidal attempt is a "cry for help"
	– to provide opportunity in discussing other methods of coping with crisis rather than suicide

Strategies	Rationale
Role Function Mode − Provide therapeutic tasks according to client's capabilities and previous interests	− to prevent further self-deprecation, worthlessness − tasks may allay guilt feelings and fulfill need for punishment − promote feelings of being needed and approval − to assess concentration span and ability to perform − to stimulate mental processes − to gradually promote social interaction − to re-establish previous skills and interest − to foster sense of accomplishment
− Allow to make simple decisions	− to maintain self-esteem − to promote self-confidence in decision making − to provide opportunity in testing problem solving skills − to increase positive aspect of self-concept and foster independence − assist to accept responsibility and set goals for self − guide in making decision, if unable, make decision for client indirectly. Collaborative decision making is more effective − to rebuild self-respect
Interdependence Mode − Inform client and family of treatment plan	− to foster trust and confidence in health team members − to provide opportunity for family to express concerns and reactions towards suicide − to prevent further isolation and alienation, eliminate anxiety to both client and family − to promote continuity of treatment plan and co-operation between family and team members during and after hospitalization
Interdependence Mode − Share with health team members the client's suicidal clues	− to institute safety precautions − to promote expression of team members reactions to suicidal act − to maintain continuity of safety measures
− Inform team members of client's responses to treatment plan	− to evaluate effectiveness and side effects of treatment − to determine other physiological malfunctions
− Determine the need for further referral to other health disciplines and community agencies	

EVALUATION

– Assess response of client to treatment plan

– Evaluate effectiveness of nursing interventions

– Modify the plan of care according to the changing needs of the client

– Re-assessment of the goals of plan of care

– Share and collaborate with other members of the health team the revision of the plan of care

Suggested Readings

Beck, A., *The Development of Depression: A Cognitive Model, The Psychology of Depression, Contemporary Theory and Research,* Washington, D.C. V. H. Winston, 1974

Birren, J. E. and Warner, S. K., *Handbook of the Psychology of Aging,* New York. Van Nostrand Reinhold Co., 1977

Burgess, A. W., *Psychiatric Nursing in the Hospital and Community,* 3rd ed., Englewood Cliffs, New Jersey. Prentice-Hall Inc., 1981

Farberow, N. L. and Shneidman, eds., *The Cry for Help,* New York. McGraw-Hill Book Co., 1961

Hoff, L. A., *People in Crisis—Understanding and Helping,* Menlo Park, California. Addison-Wesley Publishing Co., 1978

Kreigh, H. Z. and Perno, J. E., *Psychiatric Mental Health Nursing: Commitment to Care and Concerns,* 2nd ed., Reston, Virginia. Reston Publishing Co., 1983

Kyes, J. and Hofling, C., *Basic Psychiatric Concepts in Nursing,* 4th ed., Philadelphia. J. B. Lippincott Co., 1980

Lewinsohn, P. M. et. al, *Sensitivity of Depressed Individuals to Aversive Stimuli,* Journal of Abnormal Psychology, 1973, 81, pp. 259–263

Masserman, J. H., *Principles of Dynamic Psychiatry,* Philadelphia. W. B. Saunders, 1961

Poznanski, E. and Zrull, J. P., *Childhood Depression—Clinical Characteristic of Overtly Depressed Children,* Archives of General Psychiatry, 1970, 23, pp. 8–15

Roy, Sister C., et al, *Introduction to Nursing. An Adaptation Model,* New Jersey. Prentice-Hall, Inc., 1976

Seligman, M., *Depression and Learned Helplessness,* The Psychology of Depression, Contemporary Theory and Research, Washington, D.C. V. H. Winston, 1974

Stuart, G. W. and Sundeen, S. V., *Principles and Practices of Psychiatric Nursing,* 2nd ed. St. Louis. The C. V. Mosby Co., 1983

Topalis, M. and Aguilera, D., *Psychiatric Nursing,* 7th ed., St. Louis. The C. V. Mosby Co., 1978

Exercise 28
DEPRESSION

Duration:

Direction: Study the following situations and discuss your answers among your peer group.

Situation #1

Recall a personal incident where you had experienced a feeling state of depression.

What were your thoughts and feelings at the time?

How were these feelings overtly expressed?

Were you able to identify the causes of the depressive feeling state?

Situation #2

Three days after colostomy surgery, how would you respond to Miss Todd, age 40, who refuses to look at her colostomy?

Name at least five different responses.

State various emotional reactions that Miss Todd may be experiencing at the time.

What nursing actions can you implement to facilitate positive self-concept?

Situation #3

You are assigned to a chronic care setting where Mrs. Polonoski, a 65 year old widow, was admitted three months ago due to hip fracture, hypertension and depression. When you approached Mrs. Polonoski, the client stated: "Go away, no speak English. You nice but I no good. God take me now." During the three days you were assigned to Mrs. Polonoski, she continued to be apathetic and indifferent to you.

How do you think she is feeling at the moment?

What are the possible causes of the feelings you have stated?

What are some of your thoughts and feelings while caring for Mrs. Polonoski?

How did you behave as a result of these thoughts and feelings?

State various modes of communication that you can effectively utilize to assist Mrs. Polonoski verbalize her concerns.

Situation #4

Danny, an 18 month old boy, is admitted to the hospital isolation unit for gastroenteritis and dehydration. A few days after admission, noticeable behavioral changes have been observed.

What behavioral responses would you expect from Danny to indicate depression?

Name five nursing actions that you would implement to deal with the identified behavior and state your rationale for these nursing actions.

How would you deal with the anxieties of Danny's parents?

Exercise 29

DEPRESSION AND SUICIDE

Duration: 10 minutes

Direction: Mark T for true or F for false on the line to the left of each of the following statements:

_____ 1. Women attempt suicide more often than men.

_____ 2. Only cowards and weaklings consider suicide as an alternative.

_____ 3. Once suicidal, always suicidal.

_____ 4. Unfortunately suicide happens without warning.

_____ 5. It is better to discuss hopeful and pleasant things with a suicidal person than it is to discuss the person's suicidal intent.

_____ 6. Suicide attempts are manipulative ploys most of the time.

_____ 7. The surest way to commit suicide is to turn on the gas.

_____ 8. Tendencies toward suicide are always inherited.

_____ 9. Rich people attempt suicide more often than poor people.

_____ 10. Only psychotic persons try to kill themselves.

_____ 11. If a person talks about intending to commit suicide, he or she will not do it.

_____ 12. Suicidal persons are not usually intent on dying.

_____ 13. Suicide is rarely attempted by mentally retarded persons.

_____ 14. Suicide is seldom attempted by well educated persons.

_____ 15. The immediate suicide risk is over when improvement follows a depression.

Exercise 30

THE DEPRESSED CLIENT

Debbie, an 18 year old, single female, was admitted to an emergency department of a general hospital for attempting to slash her wrists. History revealed that Debbie has attempted suicide several times and was under psychiatric treatment for some time. Previous information revealed that the client had dropped out of school at an early age due to failure, minor insubordination, inability to get along with her classmates. It became apparent that Debbie incessantly complained of headaches, nausea and inability to sleep. She had also lost some weight and had refused to participate in any social activities.

During assessment interview, Debbie seemed reluctant to discuss herself or her home situation, manifested a dull sullen look, answered in a monosyllabic way with much effort on her part to talk. She sat quietly for long periods and appeared to be in a daze. When asked "how she is feeling now" her answers would be "Life is empty since my father left and nobody cares except him".

During her stay in the hospital, Debbie kept to herself, stayed in bed most of the time and refused to go out of her room. Nurses' notes stated that Debbie was often awake at night and continued to complain of headache and nausea. On occasion, the client was observed to be weepy, nail-biting and had a slight stutter when spoken to.

1 Identify and describe the behavioral manifestation that indicate Debbie's maladaptive responses to depression according to:
   a) physiological mode

   b) self-concept mode

   c) role function mode

   d) interdependence mode

2. Establish a nursing diagnosis and formulate a plan of care for Debbie.

3. State various behaviors that may indicate suicidal intent.

4. List five nursing actions to prevent Debbie from future suicidal attempts.

5. What are your own beliefs and attitudes toward suicide? How will these influence your nursing actions toward a suicidal client?

6. List the major classification of drugs that will most likely be prescribed for Debbie and give at least five examples.

7. Describe briefly electroconvulsive therapy, advantages and disadvantages, side effects and your nursing responsibilities.

CHAPTER 8

The Withdrawn Client

In recognizing that anxiety occurs as a result of frustration based on unfulfilled needs, one should remember that anxiety causes great discomfort and demands that action be taken to relieve the feeling. One of the ways of relieving anxiety may be uncomplicated and almost automatic. But for others who face a great many frustrations or who are unable to resolve a particular problem it can become more frustrating and the individual may be subjected to unpleasant, painful and potentially negative long term consequences of anxiety thus making him or her withdraw.

The individual who uses withdrawal as a coping style will inevitably avoid any situation that he or she perceived potentially harmful and threatening. Social living forces the individual to deal with many situations where the person becomes apprehensive and scared. It is under these circumstances where the person is unable to avoid the situation that withdrawal techniques will be employed. These evasive reactions will usually lead to failure and self-depreciation which in turn makes their use more necessary. Thus, viscious habits of response become established which lead to a complete ineffectiveness in dealing with most problems.

In addition to withdrawing physically, the individual may withdraw in a variety of psychological ways, such as reduction of ego involvement in the situation, lowering of aspiration, admitting defeat, restricting the situations with which he or she attempts to cope, curtailing energy and effort, becoming apathetic or insulating self from emotional hurt.

There are, of course, many situations where withdrawal, physical or emotional, may be the most realistic solution. However, for many individuals, withdrawal becomes a standard coping mechanism and will take precedence over any other potential alternative in given situations. As the individual learns to associate certain people or situations with frustration and hurt, he or she will withdraw rather than attempt to deal with them directly. The tendency to withdraw in the face of such situations is typically reinforced by fear. In time, these fears may generalize to involve a wide range of real or imagined fears and eventually lead to retreat from the real world.

Hostility may also be aroused since withdrawal usually involves some measure of frustration. When withdrawal is incompatible with one's idealized self-image, guilt feelings may emerge, a complicated mixture of apprehension, anxiety and self-devaluation that can greatly affect the person's self worth and distortion in perception and thinking.

When the person is functioning on the basis of a grossly distorted reality such as hallucination, delusion and bizzare behavior, he or she is said to be psychotic.

In psychotic disorders, the client manifests severe personality decompensation with marked distortion and loss of contact with reality, lowering of adaptive controls and social breakdown which leads to thoughts, feelings and actions that have not been characteristic of the individual's behavior.

Psychotic symptoms may originate from either psychological stresses or organic brain pathology or from the interaction of both. For this reason, psychotic disorders are divided into two general categories, namely, functional and organic psychosis depending on whether or not there is some demonstrable associated brain pathology. The psychosis in which these behaviors is most dramatically presented is schizophrenia.

SCHIZOPHRENIA

Schizophrenia is a term coined by Eugene Bleuler meaning "splitting of the personality" and is derived from a Greek word "schizen, to split" and "phren, meaning mind". The term is used for a group of psychotic reactions in which there are disturbances in communication, reality, relationship, thought and emotional processes, disorganization of a previous level of functioning and disturbed identity all of which lead to fragmentation of personality but without demonstrable organic disease and intellectual deficit. A characteristic insidious onset is often preceded by introversion, subdued behavior or suspicious secretiveness.

The illness often recurs, each recurrence increasing a chronic disability until a plateau is reached and consequently results in chronic invalidism which requires prolonged hospitalization.

Bleuler's concept of schizophrenia was broader than Kraepelin who called the disorder "dementia praecox" in the early days. Bleuler described the illness in terms of primary symptoms commonly referred to as four A's: ambivalence, disturbed affect, autism and loose association, and the secondary symptoms which constitute the basic defensive framework of the disease process.

Ambivalence refers to the presence and exaggeration of two opposing emotions, attitudes or wishes for the same person, goals or situations, for example, the expression of love and hate toward an object, vacillation in making decisions which are commonly manifested in the client's responses, extreme compliance or negativism.

Disturbance of affect usually take the form of flatness, bluntness, shallowness, absence of affect and inappropriate feeling tone and responses. There is lack of emotional feeling tone or an emotional response that is opposite of a normal reaction together with monotone voice and expressionless face. For example, a client may greet bereavement with laughter or indifference, or he may giggle as serious aspects of his condition are discussed. There may also be uncanny feeling of being of oneness with the universe, or changes in bodily functions or parts which are manifested through nihilistic delusions.

Autism is a form of thinking characterized by self-absorption, fantasy and day dreaming that substitute for reality. Ideas are distorted and the client is preoccupied with inner thoughts. These disturbances are frequently manifested through highly personalized language which are coined and understood only by the client together with evidence of rocky movements, banging of head and an imaginary world created by the client.

Loose association is another term for derailment which refers to a disturbed thinking process and thought content. The pattern of spontaneous responses in which thoughts to be expressed are changed and directed to other ideas that are completely unrelated making the speech pattern seem unintelligible to others. These are commonly displayed by the client's illogical sequence of responding, interpretation of statements literally, blocking, circumstantiality and the like.

The secondary symptoms of schizophrenia are defenses in attempt to halt the disintegration process of the illness or attempts at restitution through the use of defense mechanism of denial, projection, regression and depersonalization.

The use of denial can be observed either by becoming overly active and excited as in the case of catatonic furor or by denying the loss of the outside world through catatonic stupor.

The defense mechanism of projection is utilized to maintain ego integrity by blaming others for own difficulty and attributing one own's unacceptable desires to others. Such thoughts and feelings from the client's unconsciousness that are projected onto someone are directed back to ownself and in turn make up for the delusion and hallucination which are typical of the disease process. Delusions are false beliefs which are out of proportion with the client's level of knowledge and culture. There are many examples of false beliefs or delusions frequently seen in schizophrenia and the most common ones are: persecutory delusion in which the client believes he is being pursued by someone else and this explains away one's failures to achieve; grandiose delusion, a feeling of superiority and omnipotence which counteracts feelings of inferiority and inadequacy and somatic delusions which are false beliefs about the client's body functioning. Hallucinations, on the other hand, are false sensory perceptions in the absence of external stimuli where the client perceives through one of his or her sensory organs something that does not really exist in reality. It may involve any of the five senses but the one most common in schizophrenia is auditory hallucination. Hallucination and delusions have similar dynamic functions, that is the projections of undesirable impulses, unacceptable desires, unbearable guilt and wishful thinking. The most common hallucinations are auditory hallucinations which is evidenced in hearing voices and conversation with God that may be pleasant or unpleasant and frequently associated with sexual and religious connotation; visual hallucination in which the client sees unreal sights; gustatory hallucination where a client may taste something that is not really present in the mouth; olfactory hallucination is the smelling of some foul unusual odor while tactile hallucination is feeling of objects in the body which do not exist.

The defense mechanism of regression is used against the primary process by going back into an infantile level of behavior where the needs were easily met and this return to a lower level of functioning attempts to relieve anxiety.

The use of depersonalization is displayed through the feelings of strangeness and unreality about self and the environment, reflecting loss of ego boundaries and difficulty in differentiating the two, for example, client sees others as an extension of own self.

Once the person is diagnosed as schizophrenia, the client's behavior is further categorized into five major types which is demonstrated by the table that follows.

THEORIES OF SCHIZOPHRENIA

Whatever specific view of the causation of schizophrenia is endorsed, the etiology of schizophrenic reactions are still far from clear. Several theories have been advanced in an attempt to understand the process but it would seem that there are multiple causative factors operating in the formation of disease. In some instances, biological factors seem quite significant while in other instances, the psychological or sociocultural dominate the etiological pattern.

Types	Maladaption Reaction	Basic Dynamics
1. Disorganized	- shallow, inappropriate emotional responses - bizzare behavior, giggling, silliness, childish, unpredictable, grimacing - delusion but not systematized - hallucination - extreme withdrawal	- severe personality disintegration with fragmented thoughts - loss of identity - withdrawal from social contact
2. Catatonic	- conspicuous motor behavior with either generalized retardation (stupor) or hyperactivity (excitement) - bizzare posture	- client momentarily overwhelmed by problems and struggling desperately to find relief
3. Paranoid	- delusion of persecution - hallucination with constant hostility - delusion of omnipotence, remarkable talents and high social status - passivity	- an attempt to maintain ego integrity by projecting blame on others; compensate for inadequacies
4. Undifferentiated	- prominent psychotic symptoms cannot be classified into one category due to mixture of other features	- an attempt to protect self from failure by projection - client is overwhelmed by reality that delusions are not well systematized. Secondary symptoms are not yet well established.
5. Residual	- social withdrawal - emotional blunting - eccentric behavior - inconspicuous delusion or hallucination	- partial remission of the disease but still maintain some schizophrenic features without acute psychotic signs.

Figure 8.1 Summary Chart of Schizophrenia

A. Biological Theories

The biological theories include the genetic predisposition which was reflected in the studies that show if one pair of identical twin has a severe form of schizophrenia, 85% of the other twin will develop the disease. In fraternal twins of the same sex, the correlation is about 15%. Similarly, the children of schizophrenic parents are more likely to develop the illness and the expectancy rate being 16% if only one parent is schizophrenic and 40% if both parents are schizophrenic. This is the strongest evidence of genetic basis but there is no definite theory of the mode of inheritance except for hereditary predisposition.

Many biochemical anomalies and possibilities have been reported based on increasing knowledge of brain biochemistry and psychopharmacology. It has been theorized that defect in the metabolism of the indolamine serotonin will result in production of hallucinogenic substance; transmethylation hypothesis postulates that since many hallucinogens are methylated substance, an accumulation of methylated substance might occur in schizophrenics; and the dopamine hypothesis states that schizophrenia is assumed to reflect a defect in dopamine-mediated brain system which result in depleted brain catecholamine.

B. Psychological Theories

From a developmental point of view emerges several theories to illustrate the psychogenic indicators of risk factors. Bleuler emphasized the role of frustration and conflict and since then other experts focused on early traumatic childhood experiences, parental role, pathological family setting and disorganization and the effects of these on the formative years of growth and development. Other investigators have drawn on communication theory suggesting repeated exposure to double-bind experiences will make the potential client perceive the entire environment as a double-bind. Freud emphasized the role of sexual regression in the development of the illness while Sullivan suggested the client's disturbed interpersonal relationship rather than the intrapsychic factors.

C. Sociocultural Theories

Studies have pointed out the occurrence of schizophrenia in various cultures and societies and while it occurs in the same general forms, it is noted that sociocultural factors influence the incidence, type of reactions and particular symptoms. Underprivileged areas of big cities have high density populations of schizophrenics for reasons either because they are socially and economically incompetent or these areas breed schizophrenics because of population with severe socioeconomical problems and high incidence of broken homes which places limitations on achievement of fundamental needs.

Childhood Schizophrenia

There is an appreciable overlapping in abnormalities of a psychological nature among children and theories have explored these difficulties by differentiating childhood schizophrenia and infantile autism.

Despite scientific advances, abnormal child psychology remains less well developed than that in the adult field.

The following table will illustrate the several features of the differences of childhood schizophrenia and infantile autism.

Childhood Schizophrenia	Infantile Autism
Abnormalities may be present and detected as early as 1-2 years of age	Clinical picture is obvious from 1-18 months
Clinical degrees of abnormal behavior becomes full blown between the ages of 7-10 years	Appear normal in physical appearance from birth Condition becomes progressive
Highly vulnerable to threat and extreme sensitiveness to stimulus which results in withdrawal	Totally unresponsive to stimulus or human contact
Whimpering and crying most of the time	Lack of affect
Hypersensitivity, erractic behavior, severe or persistent colic, difficulty in feeding	Grossly insensitive to pain Preoccupation with inanimate objects
Non-communicative but awareness is present Lack of parental attachment	Non-communicative and no awareness of outside world; subjective thinking Severe social isolation and marked alienation
Exaggerated fearfulness and tension	Self-mutilating behaviors, i.e. head-banging, hand biting May be interpreted as mental retardation

Figure 8.2 Difference Between Childhood Schizophrenia and Infantile Autism

ASSESSMENT
THE WITHDRAWN CLIENT

Physiological Mode	Self-Concept Mode	Role Function Mode	Interdependence Mode

– hallucination
– delusion
– speech: poverty of content
    illogical
    incoherent
    repetitive
    circumstantial
    mutism
    flight of ideas
    autism
    neologism
– increased motor activities as in catatonic furor; impulsive
– decreased motor activities as in catatonic stupor
– poor muscle tone due to lack of desire to be active
– sleep pattern disturbances
– appetite may be decreased due to suspicious nature of being poisoned
– poor eating habits, i.e. may become obese or undernourished
	– dishevelled physical appearance and poor personal hygiene
	– unable to separate self from outside environment (loss of ego boundaries)
	– disturbed body image and loss of identity
	– bizzare behaviors, i.e. grimacing, mannerism, stereotyped postures
	– excessive pre-occupation with religion, sex, identity and somatic complaints
	– suspicious
	– angry
	– fearful
	– apathy
	– ambivalent
	– guilt
	– inappropriate emotional responses
	– loss of interest in self, others and environment
		– disturbed perception of role expectation
		– no motivation
		– impaired routine daily functioning
		– excessive concern for autonomy
		– negative and resistive to role expectation
		– inadequate in role function
		– cannot relate to others
		– no problem solving skills
			– suspicious
			– argumentative
			– violent or aggressive
			– negativistic
			– assaultive
			– no emotional involvement with others; indifferent to environment
			– cannot relate and uncomfortable with relationship
			– negative to suggestions

Physiological Mode	Self-Concept Mode	Role Function Mode	Interdependence Mode
– selective food intake due to chemotherapy – constipation is common due to use of major tranquilizers	– inappropriate use of defense mechanisms, i.e. denial, projection, regression, depersonalization, introjection – persecutory or grandiose judgement		

PLANNING AND IMPLEMENTATION

Strategies	Rationale
Physiological Mode – Orientate to reality	– to prevent from harming self and others as client may become impulsive and destructive due to auditory hallucination – to interrupt pattern of hallucination – to divert beliefs in hallucination as reality – to encourage contact with real persons and activities thus preventing further withdrawal and creation of fantasy world – to distinguish between self and external environment due to loss of ego boundaries – to convey sense of security and acceptance – to prevent regression
– Do not reinforce delusion	– to assist in differentiating between reality and false beliefs – to encourage recognition of delusion as such – to provide interaction on the basis of reality – to explore other ways of dealing with feelings of low self esteem, anxiety, threats, and so forth, rather than the use of delusion – to decrease anxiety thus reducing the need for delusion – delusions are coping styles utilized by clients – to prevent regression – to restore functioning at an optimum level
– Use simple statements when talking to client	– to facilitate understanding and avoid misinterpretation of topics being discussed, thereby reducing anxiety – due to alteration in the senses, client usually misinterprets words, situations, behavior of others – to assist client relate at a level of his or her understanding and facilitate ability to converse – to provide opportunities for verbal expressions – to decrease threat of self expression – to gain attention of client especially during the hallucinatory process – attention span is short that comprehension is limited or due to preoccupation

Strategies	Rationale
– Plan regular activities	– to establish and maintain physical state of homeostasis
	– activities help client remain in contact with others
	– to improve motivation and prevent further withdrawal
	– to increase self-esteem through participation
	– to prevent regression as client commonly refuses to engage in activities
	– to provide opportunities to channel aggressive and impulsive tendencies
	– to establish healthy patterns of nocturnal sleep
– Provide a quiet environment	– to decrease mounting tension that may lead to extreme agitation and restlessness
	– to promote rest and sleep
	– to prevent further environmental threats especially if client is hallucinating
– Monitor food and fluid intake	– to maintain adequate nutrition and hydration
	– alteration in physical homeostasis may ensue, i.e. nausea, gastric irritation, thirst, fatigue, as a result of chemotherapy
	– to ensure adherence to prescribed food, i.e. some food may be contraindicated due to chemotherapy
	– to observe eating habits thus preventing unbalanced diet
– Decrease suspicion regarding food intake	– due to suspicious behavior of the client, he or she may refuse to eat for fear of being poisoned
	– persecutory delusion may hinder the client to eat for punitive reasons
	– Nihilistic delusions may prevent client to ingest food based on belief of non-existent gastrointestinal organs
– Monitor elimination pattern	– to establish bowel regularity as constipation frequently occurs due to use of major tranquilizers
	– to maintain hydration due to polyuria
Self-Concept Mode – Assist client with personal hygiene	– lack of motivation contributes to negligence of personal activities of daily living
	– to increase self-esteem and self worth
	– to convey interest and caring
	– to help client meet basic needs
– Spend time with client	– to establish contact as client has extreme difficulty relating to others
	– to provide for interaction thus assisting him or her re-establish ego boundaries
	– to establish rapport and trusting relation
	– to provide opportunities for close observation and early intervention before behavior becomes uncontrollable
	– to provide positive feedback and emotional support
	– to convey interest, caring and acceptance of behavior

Strategies	Rationale
– Do not reinforce delusion	– see physiological mode
– Intervene with hallucinatory process	– see physiological mode, orientation section
– Provide a safe and secure environment	– to establish daily routine activities to promote security as client becomes easily threatened with changes
	– to maintain safe environment for client and others in the event that behavior becomes too bizzare and disturbing to others and self
	– to set limits on behavior as client is unable to control own behavior
	– to provide for closer observation and evaluation of client's behavior and functioning
	– client may function in an optimum level within a controlled environment
	– to provide safety measures in the event of suicide in response to hallucination
– Assist client express present feelings and experiences	– see chapter VII, Depression, section on planning and implementation, "assist client to verbalize"
	– to prevent further withdrawal and regression
	– to assist handling distressful feelings due to hallucination
	– to orientate client to reality
	– to promote interaction based on reality
Role Function Mode – Teach simple skills	– to re-establish some sense of role expectation
	– to evaluate the level of optimum level of functioning
	– to provide opportunities for assuming responsibility in activities of daily living
	– to ensure accomplishment of assigned tasks as client has difficulty in concentration and is preoccupied
	– to increase self-esteem and self worth
– Plan activities with client	– promote feelings of being needed and approval
	– to foster sense of accomplishment
	– to maintain healthy aspect of the behavior
	– to evaluate interest
	– to increase motivation
	– to facilitate interaction with others
	– to provide situations to test problem solving skills

Strategies	Rationale
– Health Teach re Drug Therapy	– to prevent non-compliance to drug therapy and avoid exacerbation of illness
Interdependence Mode – Provide opportunity for social interaction	– to promote feeling of belonging
	– to re-establish social skills
	– to facilitate interaction with others
	– to prevent further isolation and alienation as client tends to become quickly dependent on staff
	– to learn how to behave in a socially acceptable way
	– to maintain sexual identity through socialization process
– Encourage participation in group activities	– same as above
	– to promote active participation in treatment modalities

EVALUATION

– Assess client's responses to nursing interventions and treatment modalities

– Modify and propose alternative approaches to treatment plan and nursing interventions

Suggested Readings

Burgess, A. W., *Psychiatric Nursing in the Hospital and the Community*. 3rd ed., Englewood Cliffs. Prentice Hall Publishing Co., 1981

Hays, J. S. and Larsen, K. H., *Interacting with Patient*. New York. MacMillan Co., 1969

Kreigh, H. and Perko, J., *Psychiatric and Mental Health Nursing: Commitment to Care and Concern*. 2nd ed., Reston, Virginia. Reston Publishing Co.,—A Prentice Hall Co., 1983

Kolb, L. C., *Noyes' Modern Clinical Psychiatry*. 10th ed. Philadelphia. W. B. Saunders Co., 1982

Kyes, J. and Hofling, C. *Basic Psychiatric Concepts in Nursing,* 4th ed., Philadelphia. J. B. Lippincott Co., 1980

Rutter, M, *Childhood Schizophrenia Reconsidered*. J. Autism Childhood Schizophrenia, 2, 315–337, 1972

Stuart, G. W. and Sundeen, S. V., *Principles and Practice of Psychiatric Nursing*. 2nd ed., St. Louis. The C. V. Mosby Co., 1983

Topalis, M. and Aguilera, D., *Psychiatric Nursing*. 7th ed., St. Louis. The C. V. Mosby Co. 1978

THE WITHDRAWN PATIENT

Paul B., an 18 year old single male patient, was admitted to the hospital by his parents. According to his parents, Paul displayed tremendous change in his personality two years ago and he became progressively worse until the time of admission. He spent a great deal of time wandering aimlessly, refused to go to work or attend school, was very uncooperative at home, sleeping most of the day and listening to the radio all night.

About three months ago, Paul became frankly delusional, stating that "people are out to get me". He became extremely withdrawn, could not take care of himself and became emaciated due to refusal to eat for fear of being poisoned.

During interview, Paul stated "I can predict things that are going to happen". He heard voices saying, "There goes the hockey hero" and stated that his problems are due to a misunderstanding between him and his father.

Upon admission, the nurse observed that Paul was grimacing, appeared haggard-looking, affect was shallow and was quite aloof and indifferent to the environment.

History revealed that Paul's relationship with his parents consisted of getting them to take care of him and make decisions for him, particularly his mother.

1. Assess Paul's behavior and past history according to:
   a. physiological mode

   b. self-concept mode

   c. role function mode

   d. interdependence mode

2. State your nursing diagnosis and formulate a plan of care for Paul.

3. State various behaviors that may indicate the following:
   a. suspiciousness

   b. hallucination

c. delusion

4. List five nursing actions for Paul when he is:
   a. hallucinating

   b. delusional

   c. withdrawn

   d. suspicious

5. Describe briefly the following treatment modalities:
   a. Remotivation therapy

b. Reality orientation

c. Group therapy

d. List the major classification of drugs that will be most likely prescribed for Paul and give some examples of each.

Exercise 32

MALADAPTIVE BEHAVIOR I

Duration: 10 minutes

Direction: Match Column I with Column II

COLUMN I	COLUMN II

COLUMN I

A. Absence of psychical feeling

B. Misinterpretation of stimulus

C. Distractibility

D. Ruminative thinking

E. Loss of ego boundaries

F. Disorder without presence of brain pathology

G. Concern about physical health

H. Disorder with structural brain changes

I. Attribution of undesirable traits to others

J. Sensory perception in the absence of external stimulus

K. Return to lower level of functioning

L. Relating of a situation with minute details

M. Unconscious projection of incidence as if it has reference to oneself

N. Reaction characterized by silly, bizzare behavior and inappropriate responses

O. State of indifference

P. Presence of two opposing feelings

Q. Feeling tone

R. Motionless position

S. False belief

T. Coining of words

COLUMN II

_____ 1. Autism

_____ 2. Delusion

_____ 3. Affect

_____ 4. Ambivalence

_____ 5. Depersonalization

_____ 6. Apathy

_____ 7. Circumstantiality

_____ 8. Illusion

_____ 9. Hallucination

_____ 10. Projection

_____ 11. Waxy flexibility

_____ 12. Somatization

_____ 13. Functional psychosis

_____ 14. Flight of ideas

_____ 15. Organic psychosis

_____ 16. Ideas of reference

_____ 17. Disorganized type

_____ 18. Passivity

_____ 19. Neologism

_____ 20. Regression

CHAPTER 9

The Hyperactive Client

The term Affective Disorders refers to a mental disorder in which the fundamental disturbance is in the mood and the condition manifests itself into two distinct and contrasting forms, that is, depression which was discussed in Chapter VII and the manic phase which is characterized by hyperactivity in varying degrees and duration.

The first attempt to understand mania was introduced by Abraham in 1911 who was the first analyst to compare normal grief with depression. While working out his ideas on depression he discovered that mania appeared to be a polar opposite and the dynamic considerations of this condition were quite similar to those of depression. Meanwhile Kraepelin categorized all these behavior manifestations into one syndrome called Manic-Depressive Psychosis, the term commonly used in the previous classification of psychiatric disorders. At present, the disorder is classified as Major Affective disorders, bipolar disorder and the different types of reactions are further classified into subtypes. For further information of the different types, refer to Appendix A, DSM III official classification.

There is now evidence to indicate that clients suffering from this disorder have both the manic and depressive illnesses at different times which is called bipolar, and while others just have the depression and is referred to as unipolar. Depressions are often preceded or followed by brief episodes of hypomania and the converse is equally true of the manic phase which is often punctuated by periods of weeping and sadness. The manic phase is in many respects the mirror of its depressive counterparts.

The hyperactivity describes the overall acceleration of mood and psychomotor activities in which the client becomes highly active in all spheres of functioning; albeit maladaptive, from normal adaptation.

The behavior is easily recognized because of overactivity, distractibility, incessant speech patterns, grandiosity and lack of inhibition. The client may appear extremely confident with an ego that knows no boundaries. Accompanying these feelings of magical omnipotence and great self-esteem there is a lack of guilt and shame. There is denial of danger in a realistic sense and the client may be overinvolved in social activities and appear as the gregarious life of the party. Excessive planning in terms of ambitions without insight into possible consequences often lead to irresponsible enterprises and excessive spending of money.

The client may function for days without sleep, constantly active and quickly changing from one enterprise to another. In spite of the characteristic behaviors the condition is often misinterpreted due to similarities although different from schizophrenic reactions. For example, the hyperactive client's speech, ideas, emotions and behaviors may have become too disorganized like the withdrawn client but the exuberance, zest and jovial mood of the hyperactive client is absent in a withdrawn individual. Unlike the withdrawn client, the total functioning is less bizzare and distorted and there is better integration of self-system.

Despite the liability of recurrent illness or attacks, the hyperactive clients are endowed with unusual drives and creative abilities and do achieve success in many walks of life, function well during the remission state unlike the schizophrenics.

The onset, duration, course and recovery of the bipolar illness is almost invariable. Depressive episodes are much more prevalent than the manic phase, depression being more common in females while manic episodes are equally divided between men and women. The commonest age of onset for bipolar illness is the second or third decade of life while unipolar illness may appear at any age. Once a clear diagnosis of bipolar disorders has been established further episodes are almost inevitable and the condition tends to get more frequent with increasing age.

THE HYPERKINETIC CHILD

The most striking characteristics of a hyperkinetic child are the unpredictability of behavior and erratic changes in the mood which may be obvious as early as two years of age to the seventh years of life.

The child becomes hyperactive and restless, irritable and cranky, demanding, tendency to temper tantrum even for no apparent reason, negativistic, highly distractible, low tolerance to frustration and extreme attachment to parental figure which seems to be more out of fear rather than affection.

THEORIES OF BIPOLAR AFFECTIVE DISORDERS

A. Biological Theories

There are many theories with regard to the development of bipolar disorders and the recent ones subscribe to the notion of genetic components as manifested in occurrence of the condition in the same family. For example, studies have shown that about 15% of the parents, siblings and offsprings are similarly afflicted and studies of monozygotic and dizygotic twins also support the genetic point of view.

There also tends to be a systematic personality difference between unipolar and bipolar affective disorders. Those afflicted with bipolar tend to be energetic and extroverted with considerable emotional warmth while those afflicted with unipolar tend to be more introverted and with some obsessional traits. Other biological factors that have been previously studied correlate the condition with body build such as the pkynic body build, the mesomorphic type and cyclothymic personality.

Concurrent with the genetic components are some hypothesis that elation is accompanied by an increase in brain catecholamines while in depression there is depletion of both catecholamines and indoleamines in the hypothalamus and brain stem. Similarly, there are also reports based on whole body balance studies that the intracellular sodium content is abnormally high in depression and even more so in mania and these abnormalities usually disappear after recovery.

B. Psychodynamic Theories

From psychological point of view, the theory places emphasis on early childhood experiences where the client may have experienced a loss of parent where the mother's love or surrogate love is absent or directed toward somewhere else. During childhood there were evidences of parental expectation of achievement and prestige which placed great expectation on the child. Parental disapproval of the child's behavior led to oversensitiveness, competition, and envy among other siblings and even with own parents.

When demands are frustrated the child behaves in such a way to gain love and acceptance thus denying and repressing the hostility generated by the disapproving parents and this eventually leads into self-hatred and loss of self-esteem. In adult life, the client learns to counteract the hostility, limitations, frustrations and failures by projection and becoming aggressive.

An understanding of the theories of depression is fundamental to comprehension of the manic phase. For instance, hostility in depression is introjected because of guilt while hostility in the manic phase is directed toward the external environment which results in mania. Consequently, mania becomes a flight from reality with some regression and a defense of denial against the underlying depression.

Constitutional irregularities in infancy and some faulty maturational development are not uncommon in a hyperkinetic child. Central to the causative factors, however, is the social learning theory of markedly contradictory parental feelings and attitudes. There is usually evidence of schism in the family, ambivalence, cyclical moods and inconsistent approach to the child that is conducive to double-bind message.

ASSESSMENT
THE HYPERACTIVE CLIENT

Physiological Mode	Self-Concept Mode	Role Function Mode	Interdependence Mode

– Hyperactivity
  – agitation
  – restlessness
– Accelerated thinking pattern
  – distractibility
  – flight of ideas
  – poor concentration
  – increased perception although may not be accurate
– Poor judgement
  – no insight
  – may become disorientated
– Pressure of speech
  – loose speech pattern
  – rhyming
  – punning
  – clang association
  – incoherence
– Poor nutrition
  – appetite may be voracious to complete rejection of food due to restlessness
– Sleep and Rest
  – inability to rest and sleep due to excitability
	– fluctuation of mood, i.e. heightened emotional tone or elation to periods of depression
	– poor personal hygiene
	– inappropriate clothing
	– overly optimistic, exaggerated feelings of well-being
	– self-exalting
	– talkative, boisterous, flippant
	– irritable, impatient
	– erotic speech and behavior
	– no insight
	– no sense of guilt and shame
	– delusion of grandeur
	– hallucination may be or may not be present
	– suspicious behavior is present
		– assumes many role functions but never completes tasks
		– unreliable and lacks persistence
		– perception of role is heightened and related to sexual prowess, wealth and power
		– grandoise in role performance
		– in acute mania, is unable to function at all
			– superficial and insensitive to others
			– socially aggressive
			– intolerant of criticism
			– demanding, arrogant
			– verbally abusive
			– combative, assaultative and destructive
			– uncooperative
			– irritable
			– in hypomanic state, may be sociable and overly friendly

PLANNING AND IMPLEMENTATION

Strategies	Rationale
Physiological Mode – Provide and maintain high caloric vitamin diet and supplemental feedings	– to maintain nutrition and hydration. Client's overactivity and restlessness unables him/her to sit and eat – due to hyperactivity, client may not be aware of hunger and thirst – use of psychotropic drugs increases the need for fluid – to prevent weight loss and exhaustion due to high energy output – to prevent constipation and ensure proper elimination
– Promote rest and sleep	– to prevent fatigue and exhaustion due to hyperactivity and accelerated thought processes – to conserve energy as client is usually engaged in excessive activities for long periods, neither feeling tired or fatigued – to promote some restriction thus decreasing environmental stimuli

Strategies	Rationale
– Provide non-competitive physical activities	– to provide an outlet for excess energy
	– to channel client's energy and behavior through constructive and structured activities
	– to monitor activities that client can achieve thus decreasing feelings of failure
	– to limit group participation due to short concentration span and distractibility
	– to reduce responsiveness to environmental stimuli
– Monitor physiological signs and drug intake	– to maintain physiological homeostasis
	– to observe for signs of physical distress and exhaustion
	– to ensure effectiveness of drug therapy
	– to provide opportunities for evaluation of client's response to treatment and drug toxicity
	– to plan and implement early intervention if necessary
Self-Concept Mode	
– Provide a safe and non-stimulating environment	– to prevent physical injury to client and others since client has no awareness of danger due to defective judgement
	– to decrease environmental stimuli thus decreasing or preventing further agitation and restlessness
	– to promote safety precautions for client and others since client's quarrelsome behavior may become a source of irritation for other clients that open confrontation may ensue
– Supervise personal hygiene	– to ensure personal grooming and promote increased self-esteem
	– to encourage appropriate clothing and appearance and prevent client from becoming the object of ridicule
	– to maintain self-identity
	– to provide opportunity to observe condition of client's body, i.e. presence of bruises or other injuries
– Provide emotional support with some restriction to verbal interaction if client is in manic state	– to convey acceptance and caring
	– to reduce interpersonal stimulation
	– lengthy interaction may increase escalating agitation and tension
	– to decrease possibility of mood fluctuation as client tends to be easily irritated, impatient, boisterous and distracted
	– to prevent loss of control
	– to minimize unnecessary stimulation through interaction since speech pattern is already accelerated

Strategies	Rationale
– Set limit on client's behavior	– to provide control in the event of acting out thus making the client feel secure – to restrict client's behavior especially if client is threatening, demanding or seductive – to discourage expression of grandiose behavior – see section on delusion, Chapter VIII – to decrease unnecessary ward disturbance as other clients may lose their ability to control their own aggression if ward is disturbed – see section on Anger, Chapter V
Role Function Mode – Plan simple activities which can be accomplished	– client has short attention and concentration span that completion of tasks is difficult – to promote sense of success and counteract feelings of inadequacy and inferiority – to provide opportunity to re-focus on reality of performance without reinforcing grandiose delusion – to re-establish and maintain role function
– Assist client in performance of daily activities of living	– same as above – to provide control while encouraging independent function – to maintain self-esteem
Interdependence Mode – Minimize contact with client while in manic state but provide frequent short interaction	– to avoid misinterpretation of physical contact as "attack behavior" – to maintain physical distance between self and client for safety precaution unless external control is needed – to allow for some freedom and prevent the client from feeling of being "trapped" – to display acceptance of behavior
– Limit participation with group	– client's heightened perception of self may tend to dominate others – uncertainty of mood will make it difficult to relate to others – to decrease irritability and impulsive interaction with others – to prevent retaliation from others

EVALUATION

1. Assess effectiveness of nursing interventions and treatment plan.
2. Modify and propose alternate nursing actions.
3. Identify the factors that hinder effective interventions.

Suggested Readings

Burgess, A. W., *Psychiatric Nursing in the Hospital and the Community.* 3rd ed., Englewood Cliffs. Prentice Hall Publishing Co., 1981

Haber, J. et. al., *Comprehensive Psychiatric Nursing.* 2nd ed., New York. McGraw Hill Book Co.,—A Blakiston Publication, 1982

Kreigh, H. and Perko, J., *Psychiatric and Mental Health Nursing: Commitment to Care and Concern.* 2nd ed. Reston, Virginia. Reston Publishing Co., A Prentice Hall Co., 1983

Kolb, L. C., *Noyes' Modern Clinical Psychiatry.* 10th ed., Philadelphia. W. B. Saunders Co., 1982

Stuart, G. W. and Sundeen, S. J., *Principle and Practice of Psychiatric Nursing.* 2nd. ed., St. Louis. The C. V. Mosby Co., 1983

Taylor, C. M., *Mereness Essential's of Psychiatric Nursing.* 11th ed. St. Louis. The C. V. Mosby Co., 1982

Exercise 33

THE HYPERACTIVE CLIENT

Mrs. Paul, a 40 year old, married client, was admitted to the hospital for the third time within the last 10 years. While in the hospital, Mrs. Paul was busily flying about the laundry room, singing as she scrubbed haphazardly at her soiled underclothing. Her voice was loud and merry and gave the impression of being very confident almost to the point of daring everyone who came near her. As she worked, she splashed water all over herself and the room. When a student nurse walked into the room looking for some clothing of another client Mrs. Paul jumped as if surprised and her face became tense and rigid for an instant but almost as quickly her expression changed into laughter and smiles. She was cheerful enough and kept calling the student "dearie". She started to talk in a rapid tone of voice about many and varied topics.

Throughout the afternoon Mrs. Paul, wearing a gaudy yellow blouse and red flowered skirt with smeared rouge, heavy mascara and dishevelled hair, could be seen in every corner of the unit, agitated, talking incessantly to anyone she met about her famous exploits and many projects, singing loudly and insisting that she is a night club singer. She frequently became irritated when none of the clients would believe her and would become sarcastic. She often refused lunch and dinner because of her "rehearsals", hardly slept during the night and would occasionally demand a bath at four o'clock in the morning and order chinese food for the staff nurses.

Mr. Paul described his wife as an energetic, outgoing, friendly and hard working wife and mother when the client is relatively well. The first onset of the illness occurred after the birth of their only daughter who is now eleven years old.

1. Establish a nursing diagnosis based on Mrs. Paul's behavior and formulate a plan of care according to:
   - physiological mode

   - self-concept mode

   - role function mode

   - interdependence mode

2. Describe the behavior of a hyperactive client experiencing:
   a. hypomania

   b. acute mania

   c. delirious mania

3. Identify some defense mechanisms utilized by Mrs. Paul.

4. List the common types of treatment modalities that may be prescribed for Mrs. Paul.

5. Differentiate the type of communication techniques you would utilize for Mrs. Paul as compared to a withdrawn client.

MALADAPTIVE BEHAVIOR II

Duration: 10 minutes

Direction: Match Column I with Column II

COLUMN I	*COLUMN II*
a. hypomania	_____ 1. extreme and unstable feeling of joy
b. unipolar	_____ 2. exaggerated sense of well-being
c. bipolar	_____ 3. fragmented continuous verbalization in response to stimuli
d. flight of ideas	_____ 4. uninhibited, energetic, good humor and easily frustrated state
e. circumstantiality	_____ 5. inclusion of irrelevant and non-essential details in speech
f. clang association	_____ 6. affective disorder characterized by recurrent depressive phase
g. euphoria	_____ 7. argumentative, sarcastic, boastful and demanding
h. elation	_____ 8. affective disorder characterized by alternating episodes of mania and depression
i. mania	_____ 9. associative thought disturbance often exhibited in rhyming and punning
j. labile mood	_____ 10. unexpected and unprovoked change of feelings

CHAPTER 10

The Anxious Client

As discussed in chapter V anxiety is a universal common experience in the adaptation of an individual which can either be a signal of danger mobilizing the person's coping mechanism in reaction to a threat or it can become a symptom of a more deep seated psychological tension and conflict. To be consistent with our awareness that anxiety is the foundation for understanding all forms of maladaptive behaviors it is suggested to review the chapter on anxiety.

In the Diagnostic and Statistical Manual of Mental Disorders (DSM III–1980) the disorders that were formerly known as psychoneurosis or neurosis are now included and classified under various categories, namely: anxiety disorders; somatoform disorders; affectives disorders; dissociative disorders and psychosexual disorders.

The intent of the inclusion of these classifications in this chapter lies in the fact that it is set within the context of anxiety and the subsequent coping behaviors. Clients suffering from any of these disorders usually seek medical or psychiatric attention for the purpose of relieving the distressing effects of anxiety. Thus, to avoid redundancy in nursing care, selected maladaptive behaviors like ritualism and somatization are the focal behaviors that will be given priority in the planning and implementation of nursing interventions. In this and subsequent sections an attempt will be made to present the classification of anxiety, somatoform and dissociative orders and the different types under each heading, highlighting only the descriptions of each type.

I. Anxiety Disorders

Anxiety disorders arise as a reaction to an individual's unsuccessful efforts and attempt to compromise in dealing with the underlying needs and repressed emotional conflicts of the individual. Anxiety is the central force in these disorders and it is dominated chiefly by the symptomatic expression of anxiety or the defenses by which the ego tries to control the anxiety. The person is not aware of the relationship between the symptoms and underlying conflicts and the defenses utilized by the individual are not always satisfactory thus producing maladaptive behaviors such as phobia, obsession or compulsion from which the person is attempting to seek relief against the effect of anxiety. In other words, utilization of anxiety as a danger signal has been destroyed making the individual unable to locate the sources of apprehension and the client experiences unbearable distress, irrational impulse and bizzare thoughts as a consequence of disorganized effort. Anxiety then continues to escalate, becomes generalized and diffused and attaches itself into an incidental event or object in the environment.

Types:
1. Phobic disorders (phobic neurosis)
   – characterized by unrealistic fears that are unjustified by the object or events which prompted the fear. The inner tension is symbolized and attached to an external object. The disorder is dominated by persistent avoidance behavior which is secondary to the irrational fear of a specific object, activity or situation, i.e. agoraphobia, social phobias and simple phobias.
2. Anxiety states (anxiety neurosis)
   – is a group of reactions with varying degrees of anxiety that reflect differences in the duration and intensity of the experience. The various types of anxiety states are:
   a. Generalized anxiety disorders: is the most common type of the anxiety states and it is characterized by prolonged periods of moderate degree of anxiety with diffused, generalized apprehension and distress without any obvious behavior that is similar to phobias and compulsions.

    b. Panic disorders: a condition characterized by presence of gross disorganization, overwhelming feeling of terror that result in bizarre and irrational behaviors. It is often associated with feelings of impending doom and the reaction usually lasts for a few hours or at the most, one to two days only.

3. Obsessive-compulsive disorders
   – are characterized by recurrent and persistent ideas and thoughts while compulsions are repetitive acts that are ritualistic. The tension is controlled, symbolized and discharged through a series of repetitive thoughts and acts.

II. Somatoform Disorders

    The concept of somatoform disorders are reflected through the use of physical symptoms for which there is no demonstrable or physiological malfunctioning. Instead, there are positive evidences that the physical symptoms are associated with psychological factors. The physical symptoms serve to discharge the anxiety and inner conflicts which have been repressed, the energy was displaced, converted and disseminated through bodily symptoms.

Types:
1. Somatization disorders
   – condition characterized by recurrent and numerous physical or somatic complaints which are vague and exaggerated without any evidence of any physical disorders.
2. Conversion disorders (hysterical neurosis)
   – is characterized by sudden loss and alteration of physical functioning without physical basis for the symptoms, i.e. paralysis, blindness, loss of speech, deafness and so on.
   The unconscious conflict is displaced and expressed through some body part.
   Malingering, on the other hand, is the conscious simulation of illness to avoid intolerable situations or responsibilities.
3. Psychogenic pain
   – is characterized by the presence of prolonged and severe pain in the absence of physical findings. It is similarly related to conversion disorders in that both have a primary gain which is the relief of anxiety and the secondary gain of gaining support from the environment and the decrease of motivation to recovery for avoidance purposes.
4. Hypochondriasis
   – is characterized by chronic state of fatigue and persistence of medically undiagnosed aches and pains. The physical symptoms are employed as a means of controlling others, to make others feel guilty, avoidance of responsibilities through illness and rationalization of inadequacies.

III. Dissociative Disorders

    Closely linked to phobia and conversion, dissociative disorders are characterized by varieties of dissociation which may include expression of estrangement from self and environment to a more profound amnesia of the past and multiple personality.

Types:
1. Psychogenic amnesia
   – is the sudden failure or loss of memory of the past and identity that usually last for a few days only. As the term implies, there is no underlying organic pathology and should not be associated with memory loss of organic brain disorders.
2. Psychogenic Fugue
   – is a form of amnesia that occurs in conjunction with a flight or change from usual environment and the client assumes a new identity, forgetting the original name and assumes a different name. There is no recollection of the past and the individual may appear quite normal to others.
   It is more common during wartime or during occurrence of natural disasters.

3. Multiple personality
   - is a dissociative disorder where the client's psychic makeup is re-organized into two distinct functioning personalities. The primary or normal self is the dominant personality with sudden transition to another personality which is usually opposite to the primary character.
4. Depersonalization
   - is an experience characterized by a trance-like state where the client senses familiar objects and events as strange and/or may view ownself as unreal or unknown.

THEORIES

It is quite evident that there is no single causation for anxiety, somatoform and dissociative disorders, even for clients with similar maladaptive behaviors. Moreover, sources of anxiety will differ from client to client and their varied reactions to the sources of anxiety may take precedence from time to time.

The etiology of these disorders of which anxiety is the central focus are numerous lending themselves to various theories. Biological and genetic factors do not claim any significance or major role in the etiology. Antecedent and concurrent theories relate causation of these disorders to psychogenic and social factors.

The antecedent theories represent anxiety in terms of the effect of early childhood development where there is long dependency on the mother and/or disturbed child-mother relationship which disrupted the child's coping mechanisms particularly in dealing with threats and fears. Consequently, intrapsychic impulses are repressed and reactivated during adult life even in the presence of insignificant stimulation. The reactivation of these repressed feelings and past memories stirred up variety of associated secondary thoughts and impulses which became the primary stimulus that threatened the individual.

Although there is loss of control and functioning to a certain degree during the episodes of these disorders, the eruptions of these behaviors often serve as a useful coping for the person. By discharging the hidden and pent-up emotions although maladaptive, inner tensions are released and the client feels the relief.

Concurrent thinking relates causation to social and cultural factors and the strategies that clients utilize to cope with the distress. There is emphasis on the long history of social learning experiences that have shaped the person's personality development and patterns. For example, passive-dependent personalities are more prone to phobias; clients who utilize physical symptoms and hypochondriacal strategies have usually been accustomed to manipulate others and rationalize their inadequacies through the use of these behaviors; and clients who engage in ritualistic behaviors have been taught complete conformity and propriety.

The influence of culture has maximized the development of these disorders since maladaptive behaviors may also be shaped by the institution, tradition and values of social living. One of the problems a person is faced with today is the phase of social changes and the dehumanizing effect of modern-day society which become a psychological threat in addition to the existing intrapsychic conflicts.

Assessment

The section on Anxiety in Chapter 5 will be utilized throughout the assessment process of this section. Please refer to this section for nursing intervention of a client who is anxious.

As previously stated in this chapter, specific behaviors related to ritualistic and somatization behaviors are the only disorders that will be addressed.

ASSESSMENT
THE CLIENT WITH RITUALISTIC BEHAVIOR

Physiological Mode	Self-Concept Mode	Role Function Mode	Interdependence Mode
– see anxiety section – repetitive motor activities, i.e. hand washing, posturing, refusal to touch door knobs, and so on – persistent, unwarranted thoughts, i.e. religious preoccupation, sex and so on. Delusion may be present – Sleep and rest (see – Elimination } section on anxiety	– see section on anxiety – over-emphasis on cleanliness and neatness – self-mutilation – rigid adherence to ethical and moral standards – ambivalence – guilt feelings	– see anxiety section – excessive adherence to role function – decrease in role performance due to loss of job, status – difficulty in completion of tasks due to ritualistic routine – had difficulty in making decisions	– see anxiety section – alienation from family and others – family may reject client – isolation – ritualistic behavior may be overbearing for others that results in avoidance due to fear of others, places or events

PLANNING AND IMPLEMENTATION

Strategies	Rationale
Physiological Mode – see anxiety section	– same
– provide measures to treat existing injuries to parts of the body	– client may not realize the extent of the injuries – excoriation of skin and tissues may occur due to excessive compulsive acts, i.e. continuous scrubbing and handwashing
Self-Concept Mode – see anxiety section	– same
– project non-judgemental attitude	– client is usually aware of the purposeless activities but is unable to control the act. Judgemental and ridiculing attitude will increase anxiety thus increasing the need for ritualism.
– provide alternative methods of carrying out the ritualistic behavior	– to convey acceptance – to assist client identify alternative behavior and method of dealing with anxiety especially if ritualism is self-mutilation – attempts to eliminate compulsive acts until the client is ready will only increase anxiety – to decrease the negative effects of ritualistic behavior
– modify environment	– to facilitate carrying out of ritualism in safe settings with minimum interruption to decrease anxiety
Role Function Mode – see anxiety section	– same

Strategies	Rationale
– provide sufficient time to carry out activities	– to increase self-esteem – to allow extra time to complete tasks, ritualistic behaviors may slow down the client's performance – client may need to be verbally directed in performance
– attempt to progressively decrease the number of ritualistic performances	– to increase client's problem-solving skills
– participate in activities with client	– to prevent preoccupation with self and provide opportunities for substituting other activities other than the ritualism
Interdependence Mode – see anxiety section	
– gradually encourage participation in small group activities	– to avoid undue anxiety that may increase the need for ritualism – to provide sense of acceptance from the group – to protect the client from being the object of ridicule

EVALUATION

1. Assess the response of the client to treatment plan and nursing intervention.
2. Share and collaborate with other team members the revision of nursing approaches to provide consistency.

ASSESSMENT
THE CLIENT WITH SOMATIZATION

Physiological Mode	Self-Concept Mode	Role Function	Interdependence Mode
– see anxiety section – frequent and exaggerated physical complaints related to various organs or systems – nutrition may be impaired due to loss of appetite, nausea and vomiting – sleep and rest may be impaired due to aches and pains, insomnia fatigue – elimination may present exaggerated bowel problems – loss of sensory functions may be present, i.e. taste, olfactory	– see anxiety section – attention seeking – low frustration to stress – emotionally labile – denial of psychological problems – morbid preoccupation with health and body functions – exaggerated present physical complaints	– see anxiety section – poor employment health record – avoidance of responsibilities – extensive use of over-the-counter drugs – demanding and controlling in role performance	– see anxiety section – poor interpersonal relations – attention seeking and demanding which results in avoidance by others – lack consideration for others – repeated visits to doctor's offices – manipulative

PLANNING AND IMPLEMENTATION

Strategies	Rationale
Physiological Mode – see anxiety section	– same
– assess accurately the somatic complaints	– to validate physical complaints and the need for referral – most physical complaints are related to organs and systems – do not assume all physical complaints are hypochondriacal in nature – to determine the basis of complaints
Self-Concept Mode – spend time with client but limit the amount of time in discussion of physical symptoms	– to convey acceptance and interest on the client as a person, not on the symptoms – to promote self-esteem – to reduce isolation thus decreasing the need for physical complaints – to minimize the length of time and attention given to somatic complaints
– assist client express fears and concerns	– to provide opportunity to develop insight into somatic complaints and possible correlation to psychosocial factors – to assist client develop other methods of dealing with anxiety – to discuss client's feelings and not the physical complaints – to provide emotional support and give praise if client is able to discuss symptoms as a coping mechanism
– do not argue with the physical complaints	– physical symptoms are utilized to relieve anxiety and gain attention. If client denies the existence of psychosocial factors, anxiety will increase if somatic complaints are contradicted – clients do not consciously develop these symptoms and the complaints are real to them
Role Function Mode – involve client in activities	– to maintain self-esteem – to prevent secondary gain from the symptoms – to provide opportunity to observe client in performance of activities – to increase problem solving skills
Interdependence Mode – assist client establish support system	– to prevent isolation – to decrease the need for the symptoms if he or she feels loved and wanted

EVALUATION

1. Assess the client's responses to treatment plan and nursing interventions.
2. Provide alternative nursing actions if previous approaches are ineffective.
3. Identify why nursing actions are ineffective.
4. Identify nurses' reactions toward clients who utilize physical complaints.

Suggested Readings

Burgess, A. W., *Psychiatric Nursing in the Hospital and the Community.* 3rd ed., Englewood Cliffs. Prentice Hall Publishing Co., 1981

Haber, J. et. al., *Comprehensive Psychiatric Nursing.* 2nd ed., New York. McGraw Hill Book Co.,—A Blakiston Publication, 1982

Kreigh, H. and Perko, J., *Psychiatric and Mental Health Nursing: Commitment to Care and Concern.* Reston, Virginia. Reston Publishing Co., A Prentice Hall Co., 1983

Kolb, L. C., *Noyes' Modern Clinical Psychiatry.* 10th ed., Philadelphia. W. B. Saunders Co., 1982

Stuart, G. W. & Sundeen, S. J., *Principle and Practice of Psychiatric Nursing.* 2nd ed., St. Louis. The C. V. Mosby Co., 1983

Taylor, C. M., *Mereness Essential's of Psychiatric Nursing.* 11th ed., St. Louis. The C. V. Mosby Co., 1982

Exercise 35

THE ANXIOUS CLIENT I

Mrs. Williams, age 30, married with one child was referred to the psychiatric department from the skin clinic of a general hospital. After the consultation, Mrs. Williams was admitted to the psychiatric unit and upon admission, she displayed patches of baldness distributed all over the scalp and some bleeding due to excoriated skin from rubbing her hands. In addition, she was continuously wringing her hands and refusing to touch the door knobs for fear of germs.

According to Mrs. Williams' husband the client became steadily worse during the last six months after her holiday with her own mother. She refused to go out of the house since then, has lost some weight, complained of abdominal discomfort, weakness and fatigue, and became indifferent to their child whom she adores.

Family history revealed that the client has been a nervous, timid, shy child and was afraid of heights and insects. She was raised by an aggressive successful mother who dominated the client, making most of her decisions and even speaking for her.

Past medical history showed that Mrs. Williams has undergone psychiatric treatment for recurrent and persistent ideas of killing her mother.

1. Establish a nursing diagnosis based on Mrs. Williams' behavior and formulate a plan of care according to:
   a. physiological mode

   b. self-concept mode

   c. role function mode

   d. interdependence mode

2. Identify the defense mechanisms utilized by Mrs. Williams.

3. What specific nursing actions would you employ to assist Mrs. Williams reduce her handwashings?

4. What type of treatment modalities would likely be prescribed for Mrs. Williams?

5. Identify the contributing stimuli of Mrs. Williams' condition. Describe briefly the possible dynamics of the behaviors.

Exercise 36

THE ANXIOUS CLIENT II

Mr. Davis, age 50, married three times and with six grown up children was admitted to the hospital for the fourth time due to persistent pain and limitation of movement over his right shoulder. Medical findings revealed no demonstrable physical cause for the symptoms.

Family history showed that the client was brought up on a farm against a background of poverty and economic insecurity.

During his two previous marriages, he worked very hard but still not enough to support his family. With his third marriage however, both he and his wife managed to work quite successfully and with the financial ingenuity of the present wife, they established themselves well financially and travelled extensively all over the world.

Their marriage was apparently quite happy until two years ago when domestic quarrels frequently ensued due to financial holdings. Consequently when Mrs. Davis talked of separation, Mr. Davis started having the pain, became tremulous, sleepless, tired and irritable.

During hospitalization, the client continuously complained of pain, with some tingling sensations and numbness of the hand radiating from the shoulder. He regularly asked for PRN medications and was frequently heard saying, "These doctors don't know what they are doing and the nurses never come to give you care".

1. Establish a nursing diagnosis based on Mr. Davis' behavior and formulate a plan of care according to:
   a. physiological mode

   b. self-concept mode

   c. role function mode

   d. interdependence mode

2. Identify the defense mechanisms utilized by Mr. Davis.

3. What treatment modalities will likely be prescribed for Mr. Davis?

4. Identify Mr. Davis' behaviors that will indicate the following and describe briefly the possible dynamics of these behaviors.
   a. conversion reactions

   b. anxiety reactions

5. List at least five communication techniques that will be most effective in dealing with Mr. Davis' comments.

Exercise 37

MALADAPTIVE BEHAVIORS III

Duration: 10 minutes

Direction: Match Column I with Column II

COLUMN I

a. depersonalization

b. obsessive-compulsive

c. conversion disorders

d. phobic disorders

e. dissociative disorders

f. generalized anxiety

g. somatization

h. hypochondriasis

i. panic disorders

j. malingering

COLUMN II

_____ 1. a repressed impulse that gives rise to anxiety that is controlled by depersonalization and fugue

_____ 2. anxiety is displaced from its original source to some symbolic situation in the form of fear

_____ 3. condition characterized by anxiety that is diffused and not controlled by defense mechanism

_____ 4. repressed impulse causing anxiety is converted into functional symptoms such as paralysis and anesthesia

_____ 5. anxiety associated by persistent unwanted ideas and uncontrollable impulse to act

_____ 6. anxiety is relieved through physical symptoms

_____ 7. preoccupation with bodily functions

_____ 8. conscious simulation of physical illness

_____ 9. severe disorganization of personality due to overwhelming anxiety

_____ 10. trance-like state where the client feels estrangement from self and environment

CHAPTER 11

The Aggressive Antisocial Client

Recent years have seen much more research and interest in the subject of personality disorders. Much physical and psychological distress is now known to be based or complicated by personality make up of the individual and each psychological repercussions are reflected in behavior alteration of some kind which lead to maladaptation.

Understanding the personality characteristics and the various coping behavioral patterns can serve as a base data to grasp better the underlying process of personality disorders and the sequence through which these disorders will unfold.

The definition of personality varies according to its frame of reference or theory and they differ only in terms of their values and usefulness in predicting and controlling certain events. It can be said that personality is the sum total of the person's physical, mental and emotional make up. It is the unique organization of these characteristics that will determine the individual's typical or recurrent pattern of behavior and his or her overall internal and external pattern of responses to life adjustments. Normal and abnormal personality are relative concepts and can be represented on a continuum approach. Both are shaped by the process of growth and development but the differences in character, intensity, timing and presence of environmental influences will make some individuals learn and adopt maladaptive behaviors, while others will not. When a person displays an ability to cope with the environment in a flexible and adaptive manner that fosters personal growth and satisfaction without distortion of perception and reality, it may be said that the person possesses a normal and healthy personality. Conversely, when average daily activities, responsibilities and every day relations are responded to in a defective, irresponsible and unrealistic expectation and performance, then a maladaptive personality may be said to exist.

Personality disorders can be best described as life-long inherent maladaptive patterns of behavior and adjustment that stem primarily from faulty development and pathological trends in personality structures.

It differs from anxiety disorders and psychosis in that there is not much anxiety, personal sense of distress and distortion of reality. The disorders tend to involve patterns of aggression and acting out behaviors rather than the use of mental and emotional symptoms frequently seen in other psychiatric disorders. Most of the maladaptive traits and behaviors displayed are commonly seen in a wide variety of social context and is quite often directed toward others.

The manifestation of these behaviors are generally recognizable even at the earlier phase of growth and development, adolescence and continue throughout life.

Despite differences in the form of expression and reactions to life situations, the most common behaviors displayed are antisocial behaviors and aggression. It should be noted, however, that while antisocial and aggressive behaviors are discussed in this chapter of personality disorders, manipulations are also utilized by all individuals who maintain satisfactory adjustments in life to suit their needs. What distinguishes adaptation from maladaptive patterns is the lack of resiliency, flexibility, stability and the tendency to foster a vicious cycle of these behaviors which perpetuate difficulties in ownself and especially to others.

Patterns of aggression, on the other hand, may vary from subtle manifestation as observed in passive resistance to the more overt release of aggression through physical attacks. The aggressive impulse may be the motivational force underlying numerous behaviors such as verbal threats, gossiping, inciting others to aggress and to destruction of property. Frequent exposure to frustration will generate power of the aggressive impulse. There are individuals who cannot express aggression owing to cultural social inhibitions which forbid and block its release. Consequently, they develop a degree of anxiety which immobilizes them to the extent of being unable to act out their aggression.

Aggressive behavior may be defensive or offensive and it may be aimed to meet some need or to achieve an extrinsic reward, punish others as well as destroy. It may be active or passive, direct or indirect. There are also various types of aggression. The type commonly associated with emotional or psychiatric disorders is what some authorities refer to as angry aggression.

Anger is an emotional drive that may reinforce and heighten aggressive behavior. Although it is possible to suppress an outward show of anger, anger has mounting physiological effects and becomes a driving motivational force. When angry aggression is released, anger is reduced in its intensity. Hostility, a feeling component of some aggressive acts, is also recognizable even in subtle patterns of aggression.

There have been instances when aggressive behavior has been explained as self-assertive behavior aimed to achieve independence and autonomy, compensatory actions to overcome feelings of inferiority, testing of reality and responses of significant persons. In some instances, aggression has been interpreted as unconscious striving to meet needs for affections, recognition and power.

It is with the preceding consideration in mind that the concept of manipulative antisocial and aggressive behavior are discussed in this section. It is important to recognize that while patterns of antisocial behavior, manipulation and aggression are viewed to be especially peculiar to personality disorders, the dimension and utilization of these concepts may lend itself to be the prime focus of nursing interventions for any maladaptive behaviors previously cited and studied throughout the manual.

THEORIES

A. Hereditary Disposition

The theories that disposition to behavior may be in part rooted in genetic factors cannot be overlooked in searching for biological origins. The wide variety of overt physical traits can be found among many different personality types. The high percentage and frequency of overt hostile behavior commonly observed among members of the family suggest that constitutional disposition can be traced in the development of aggressive patterns.

Although convincing evidence is still lacking there is reason to believe among members of a family group that suggest the operation of hereditary determinants and high probability of evolving into some types of personality. These findings, however, may also reflect environmental influences and can be attributed in large measure to learning.

B. Social Learning

The logic for this theory of learning applies especially to the style of learned interpersonal behavior exhibited in these relationships. Theorists believe that such individuals received little attention and love from their parents as a child and as a consequence were deprived of the social and emotional contact necessary to learn human attachment behaviors. Similarly, parents who are limited in their capacity to experience intense emotions are likely to evoke these responses in their offsprings and the children learn to imitate the patterns of interpersonal relation to which they are exposed.

C. Early Childhood Experiences

In addition to the variety of learning experiences is the lack or intensity of stimulus enrichments which may either deprive the child of developing adequate coping skills if the parents are over protective or when the parents are over demanding that the child is forced to behave in such a way in order to secure their commendation and esteem. In other words, the child must behave according to parental expectations and demands to receive the love and affection. To achieve this goal and avoid the fear of retaliation, the child learns to manipulate others in order to elicit attention and gain approval to meet and suit his own need. These patterns of experiences did not provide depth of inner feelings so that in later life the person is unable to form and sustain satisfactory meaningful interpersonal relations.

DYNAMICS OF AGGRESSION

Bringing together the use of aggression in other mental illnesses, the following table will describe briefly the process, motivation and needs of aggressive behaviors.

TYPES OF PERSONALITY DISORDERS

To assist the learner understand the current DSM III classification of disorders formerly classified under the personality disorders, the following table will outline the diagnostic categories and describe briefly the types of disorders. For further study, refer to Appendix A.

Specific Mental Disorders	Process, Motivation, Needs
Schizophrenic disorders	Accusatory, persecutory hallucinations threaten the weak self concept and security feelings. Misinterpretation of contact approaches by others provokes fear reactions of personal harm or the removal from unreality towards reality, resulting in hostile threats or behavior actions. Aggression meets the need to ward off threats in protecting the self concept and personal security.
Bipolar disorders	Pressures of internal cravings, inferiority and insecurity feelings emerge in a flow of physical activity, verbalization, demand hostile threats toward others. Aggression meets the need to release repressed psychic, physical energies and cravings with their associated anxiety and insecurity feelings, as well as the need to gain recognition and control the environment.
Unipolar disorders	Personal preoccupation with guilt feelings over magnified past events, as well as fear of inability to control anger, resentment of feelings, provokes the turning of aggression upon the self through self-mutilating actions. Residual anger, resentment feelings may be projected upon others in the form of verbal tongue lashing, unwarranted accusations and physical resistance towards persons offering emotional support. Aggression meets the need for self-punishment, and release of anger, resentment feelings.
Personality disorders	Persistent environmental frustrations provoke immature reactions of irritability, pathologic resentment feelings expressed through temper tantrums, sometimes destructive behavior. Aggression meets the need for dependency and self-gratification.
Paranoid disorders	Persecutory delusions, fear of personal physical harm may provoke accusations towards others of plots, spying, exerting control attempts, as well as the projection of hostile impulses. Aggression meets the need to project persecutory delusions, fears, and hostile impulses.
Organic brain disorders	Loss of memory for reality and its frustration may provide periodic temperamental episodes to make self inaccessible to others. Aggression meets the need to protect self and conceal loss of environmental control and project hostile impulses to others.

Figure 11.1 Behavior Dynamics Related to Aggression

Paranoid personality disorders	Hypersensitivity, chronic long standing mistrust, suspiciousness, avoidance of intimacy, jealousy, envy
Schizoid personality disorders	Inability to form social relation, introversion, aloof, shy, distant, seclusive
Schizotypal personality disorders	Previously diagnosed as schizophrenic, schizoid personality, social isolation, peculiarities in speech, thinking, perception, mannerisms and eccentricity
Histrionic personality disorders (formerly known as hysterical)	Dramatic display of emotions, overly reactive to situations, superficial, insecure, shallow, seductive, demanding poor interpersonal relation

Figure 11.2 Personality Disorders

Figure 11.2—*Continued*

Narcissistic personality disorders	Fluctuation in relationship, self-centered, preoccupation with dreams of achievement, constantly seek admiration and attention, self-absorption, overly concerned with appearance
Antisocial personality disorders (formerly known as sociopath)	Manipulative, superficial, charming, long history of antisocial behaviors, poor employment and marital records, inability to form meaningful relation, lack of responsibility, no moral and ethical standards, often in conflict with law and authority, acting out behavior is a response to stress situation
Borderline personality disorders	Unstability of mood, impulsive behavior, acting out, episodes of intense anger, clinging relation, unpredictable self-destructive acts
Avoidant personality disorders	Although similar to schizoid personality, yearns for love and affection but is cautious about relationship unless given strong guarranties, social withdrawal, overly sensitive to rejection
Dependent personality disorders	Inability to assume responsibility for own needs, no self confidence, fear of being alone, depends on someone for meeting needs, difficulty in making decisions, belittles self
Compulsive personality disorders	Need to control, fear of mistakes, preoccupation with order, neatness, efficiency, overconcern with morals, emotional constriction, indecisiveness

ASSESSMENT
THE AGGRESSIVE ANTISOCIAL CLIENT

Physiological Mode	Self-Concept Mode	Role Function Mode	Interdependence Mode
– agitation – restlessness – insomnia – poor judgement – uncontrolled sexual impulses	– perceives self as important and powerful – easily frustrated, irritated – poorly controlled impulses, low tolerance to stress, frustration, failure – suspicious – use defense mechanisms of denial, projection, rationalization, fantasy, isolation – lack adherence to ethical and moral standards – minimal anxiety and guilt – somatization	– poor interpersonal relation – lacks responsibility – non-compliant to rules and regulations – resistive to role performance – inefficient performance due to fluctuation of moods – poor employment record – often in conflict with authority – poor marital records – manipulative – failure to learn from experiences	– manipulative – disregard for social customs and amenities – no concern for others – poor interpersonal relation – demanding, impulsive, attention seeking, uncooperative, negativistic – unable to form meaningful relation – sexual acting out – threatening and hurtful to others – irresponsible acts or behaviors which may result in unlawful actions or crimes

Strategies	Rationale
Physiological Mode – see section on Hyperactive Client, Chapter IX	
– determine the need for PRN medication, seclusion or use of physical restraints	– to prevent imminent physical aggression and acting out behavior – to provide protection and safety measures until self control is fully regained – to reduce anxiety, agitation
Self-Concept Mode – observe factors that precipitate changes in behavior	– to interrupt imminent impulsive acting out behaviors – to provide provision for client's safety and others – to recognize client's need for distance and space – to identify sources of stress, frustration and failure
– assist client to express feelings	– to encourage discussion of problems rather than act on feelings – to become aware of behaviors that cause problems – to identify controlling behaviors utilized by client and determine the purpose – to establish self-esteem and convey acceptance – to explore alternate methods of coping
– provide safe environment	– see section on Hyperactive Client, Chapter IX – to reduce environmental stress
– display non-judgemental attitude	– antisocial behaviors will evoke negative feelings from others and/or punitive responses – failure to receive approval and meet physical and psychological needs will perpetuate aggression and acting out behaviors – staff members and others may become easily irritated by client's behavior that may lead to confrontation
– set limits in frequency and length of interactions	– client is manipulative and will control interactions and monopolize conversation – to discourage irrelevant topics for discussion, i.e. yourself, other staff members or clients – to focus only on discussion of client's problems and events that led to admission
Role Function Mode – set limits on behavior	– client has no control of impulses. Setting expectations on role function will provide some control and security – to assist client become responsible for own behavior – to provide positive feedback on responsible behavior – to become aware and discuss consequences of behavior
– be consistent, kind but firm in approach	– to enforce unit and hospital policies and avoid future confrontation and arguments with client – to avoid independent changes in rules and regulations as consequence of manipulative ploys of client

Strategies	Rationale
– assist client develop appropriate problem-solving skills	– to prevent formation of dependency and demanding relation
	– problem-solving skills of client are usually unrealistic and impulsive due to poorly controlled hostilities
	– to facilitate employment skills
	– to overcome feelings of inferiority and failure
	– to develop socially acceptable behavior
– engage client in constructive activities that will interest him or her	– see section on The Hyperactive Client, Chapter IX
	– utilization of potential abilities will increase self-esteem and facilitate personal growth
	– to train client to tolerate stress
	– to prepare client for discharge
	– to ascertain client's present skills and optimum level of functioning
Interdependence Mode – assist client to establish control of acting out behavior	– to discourage inappropriate use of aggression that promotes alienation of others from client
	– to help client become aware of impulsiveness and acting behaviors as problems
	– to decrease use of acting out behavior as means for primary and secondary gains
	– to provide alternative ways of coping with stress and frustration
	– to protect client from self and others
	– to assist client accept responsibility for behaviors
	– to improve ability to delay gratification
	– to prevent rejection and isolation from others
	– to convey interest and caring
– teach client to regain control over sexual impulses	– to prevent discomfort created in others by inappropriate sexual behaviors
	– to assist client develop appropriate ways of meeting sexual needs
	– provide opportunity to discuss how to deal with sexual impulses
	– identify to client behaviors that are sexually provocative
	– provide opportunity for client to realize that sexual behaviors will not gain attention and interest from others, including staff members
	– to assist client become aware of the consequences of inappropriate sexual behaviors
– use confrontation appropriately	– to assist client work through the consequences of behavior
	– to provide opportunities for constructive ways to deal with frustration
	– to help client become aware of behaviors that cause problems
	– to avoid unnecessary and over-use of confronting acting out behavior
	– promote honesty in communications

Strategies	Rationale
– be aware of client's manipulative maneuvers	– to prevent being taken in by client's flattery and sexual provocations
	– client's superficial, charming, smooth talking and friendly ways may impede and sabotage therapeutic effectiveness of nursing actions and treatment plan
	– it is easy to believe the client because of their manipulative ploys
	– to create awareness of feelings caused by the manipulative behavior

EVALUATION

1. Assess effectiveness of nursing actions and treatment plan.

2. Identify the factors that hindered or facilitated effectiveness of treatment plan and nursing approaches.

3. Propose alternate nursing actions.

4. Analyze your own reactions and attitudes toward a client with personality, impulse control and psychosexual disorders.

Suggested Readings

Bandura, A., *Aggression: A Social Learning Analysis.* Englewood Cliffs. Prentice Hall, 1973

Burgess, A. W., *Psychiatric Nursing in the Hospital and the Community.* 3rd ed., Englewood Cliffs. Prentice Hall Publishing Co., 1981

Haber, J. et al., *Comprehensive Psychiatric Nursing.* 2nd ed. New York. McGraw Hill Book Co., A Blakiston Publication, 1982

Kreigh, H. and Perko, J., *Psychiatric and Mental Health Nursing: Commitment to Care and Concern.* 2nd ed., Reston, Virginia. Reston Publishing Co., A Prentice Hall Co., 1983

Millon, Theodore, *Disorders of Personality: DSM III: Axis II.* New York. John Wiley and Sons, 1981

Stegne, L., *The Prevention and Management of Disturbed Behavior.* Toronto, Ontario Government Book Store, 1977

Stuart, G. W. & Sundeen, S. J., *Principle and Practice of Psychiatric Nursing.* 2nd ed. St. Louis. The C.V. Mosby Co., 1983

Taylor, C. M. *Mereness Essential's of Psychiatric Nursing.* 11th ed., St. Louis. The C. V. Mosby Co., 1982

Exercise 38

THE AGGRESSIVE ANTISOCIAL CLIENT

Doug, a 28 year old male client, divorced twice, was admitted to the hospital by the police after his girlfriend telephoned the station and accused the client of beating her severely. Upon admission, Doug was under the influence of alcohol, restless, verbally abusive and was threatening to kill his girlfriend upon release from the hospital.

During the assessment interview the following day, Doug enjoyed the attention of the social worker and very quickly elicited the sympathy of the staff members by his attitude of helplessness and remorse for what he did.

Doug is the only boy in a family of six children, his father was a successful business contractor and was away most of the time. His mother was an emotional but charming woman who took great care to look after the children, especially Doug.

History revealed that since the age of 12 years, the client has been a "problem child" with a reputation for being hypersensitive, stubborn and irritable. He often indulged in temper tantrums, was suspended in school three times for misconduct and beating other classmates. He often left home without the consent of his parents, was detained in a juvenile center at the age of 15 years for truancy and theft. This pattern of behavior continued until he left school at the age of 18, got married and divorced after a year. He worked occasionally as a salesman and was often discharged shortly after due to lack of responsibility, habitual lying and seductive behavior. The client remarried again at the age of 22 and was separated after six months. No detailed explanation of the two marriages was given. Instead, he is often heard to boast about his series of affairs with older women who apparently supported him.

During his hospitalization, Doug was always well groomed and dressed, made new friends, was frequently seen socializing with other clients and appeared to be the center of attraction. He often teased the student nurses and other staff members, was cooperative and pleasant. Frequent attempts have been made by the client to get weekend passes to visit his family, who refused to have anything to do with him. When permissions have been denied, Doug would flare up, become argumentative, negativistic, and refused to participate in group therapy and other activities in the unit.

1. Assess Doug's behavior and past history according to:
   a. physiological mode

   b. self-concept mode

   c. role function mode

   d. interdependence mode

2. State your nursing diagnosis and formulate a plan of care for Doug.

3. Identify specific behaviors of Doug that will reflect the following:
   a. aggression

   b. antisocial behavior

   c. manipulative behavior

4. List the defense mechanisms utilized by Doug and explain the purpose of its usage.

5. What type of personality disorder is manifested by Doug? Describe the dynamics of this personality type.

6. Name and describe the type of treatment modality that will be likely prescribed for Doug.

7. What are the problems that you might encounter during your nurse-client interaction with Doug? Why?

MALADAPTIVE BEHAVIOR IV

Duration: 10 minutes

Direction: True and False statements

_____ 1. The great majority of antisocial behaviors lack concern and awareness for the feelings of others.

_____ 2. Absence of parental model is conducive to the production of aggressive personality.

_____ 3. Borderline personality disorders are characterized by preoccupation with orderliness and strict adherence to moral and ethical standards.

_____ 4. Parental overvaluation and indulgence contribute to the development of personality disorders.

_____ 5. It is not common to hear remarks that aggressive clients have been unmanageable, uncooperative, stubborn and undaunted by punishment during the formative years of life.

_____ 6. Antisocial behaviors are defenses against feelings of inferiority, inadequacies, and low self-esteem.

_____ 7. Aggressive individuals are often endorsed and sanctioned in our society and are frequently labeled as successful efficient workers.

_____ 8. Manipulative clients often seek therapy because of anxiety attacks, sexual impotence and marital discords.

_____ 9. One of the major focus of treatment in personality disorders is to guide the client to recognize the source and character of the disorder.

_____ 10. The most common maladaptive problems of clients with antisocial behaviors are in the area of role function and interdependence rather than the self-concept mode.

CHAPTER 12

The Client with Substance Use Disorders

The history of the use of alcohol and drugs dates far back in the early record and history of mankind. At that time, however, use of the substance was considered moral problems which resulted from lack of will power and moral weakness. It is only in the recent decades that the condition has come to be regarded as psychiatric disorders.

Scientific studies and investigations have advanced and led to the tremendous progress and understanding of the problem and its subsequent impact on the psychosocial, socio-economic aspects. The problem combines the feature of both functional and organic disorders since the initial manifestation is usually of functional impairment and terminates with some evidence of organic disorders as a result of long after effects of substance abuse and dependence.

The current DSM III states that abuse or dependence of all substance that affect the behavior and mood of a person are subsumed under the category of Substance Use Disorders, formerly termed as Addiction.

The disorder is subdivided into:

1. Substance Abuse: characterized by psychological dependence and pathological use of substance that results in social and occupational impairment.
2. Substance Dependence: in addition to the character of substance abuse, there is increase of tolerance to the substance and followed by withdrawal symptoms.

Classes of Substances delineated are:

1. alcohol
2. barbiturates, sedatives, hypnotics
3. opiates
4. cocaine
5. amphetamines
6. cannabis
7. phencyclidine
8. tobacco (not considered substance abuse disorder due to lack of intoxication syndrome)

THEORIES

Dependence on the consumption of any of the substances mentioned earlier is considered a symptom or an illness, or may be both.

Causative factors cannot be specifically identified and the cause is still unknown as there is no definite dynamic picture that fits all types. What determines the particular choice of substance abuse and dependence as mode of adjustment is also still uncertain.

Many theories regarding causation and psychopathology have been offered and most authorities believe that the chief contributing factors to the disorder are psychological in nature rather than pathophysiological. The most accepted views may be summarized as follows, namely:

1. despite the fact that there is no definite substance abuse personality type, there is sufficient evidence to indicate that the majority of clients with substance abuse disorder possess some type of personality disorders, disorders of impulse control and psychosexual disorders.

2. substance abuse is utilized to establish psychodynamic equilibrium related to unresolved emotional conflicts.

3. substance abuse is the result of a complex interaction of psychological, sociocultural, biological and possibly genetic factors. For example, the parental influence during the formative years; traumatic early childhood development particularly during the oral phase; inherited traits that produce unusual reactions and distress upon ingestion of alcohol; and the sociocultural mores and customs of a particular culture.

4. substance abuse is a means to release tension, ward off anxiety and deal with environmental stress.

ASSESSMENT
THE CLIENT WITH SUBSTANCE USE DISORDERS

Physiological Mode	Self-Concept Mode	Role Function Mode	Interdependence Mode
– blurred vision, dilated pupils – slurred, incoherent speech – hypersensitivity to light and sound – impaired memory, disorientation – visual and auditory hallucination – motor incoordination: tremors, numbness, jerky movements – restlessness, agitation – muscular and abdominal aches and pains – anorexia, dehydration, poor nutrition, weight loss – insomnia, fatigue – sexual impotency, uncontrolled sexual impulses *Withdrawal symptoms* – chills and excessive perspiration – tremors, agitation and restlessness – nausea and vomiting – anorexia – lacrimation, rhinorrhea – elevation of temperature, pulse and respiration – cardiac arrhythmias	– see section on personality disorders, Chapter XI – guilt, self doubt, low self esteem – somatization – inappropriate expression of aggression – fearful, distrustful – tend to be paranoid, overly sensitive to criticism – lack of moral and ethical standards – low tolerance for stress – impulsivity – grandiose behavior – use defense mechanisms of denial, rationalization, projection, regression – anxiety, depression – suicidal attempts	– impaired social and occupational functioning – difficulties in interpersonal relationship – marriage breakdown, verbal and physical abuse – high level of dependency although resentful of authority – accident prone on job; frequent absenteeism; frequent job changes; difficulty in completion of tasks; irresponsible performance – financial dependency – poor problem solving skills – inadequate motivation or lack of it	– see personality section, Chapter XI – impulsivity, erratic, manipulative behavior – social isolation – association with peer substance abuse users – truancy, vagrancy, theft – frequent arrest, criminal behavior – sexual promiscuity – dissatisfaction with life; unrealistic goals or lack of it

Physiological Mode	Self-Concept Mode	Role Function Mode	Interdependence Mode
– convulsion, delirium tremens – hallucinations *Complications* After prolonged use of substance, client may develop any of the following—cirrhosis of the liver, nutritional and vitamin deficiency, chronic brain damage, mental deterioration			

PLANNING AND IMPLEMENTATION

Strategies	Rationale
Physiological Mode – monitor physiological functioning	– to assess and establish level of consciousness – to establish baseline data and observation of further physical and physiological complications – to observe withdrawal symptoms as decrease or attempts to control consumption of any substance used will precipitate withdrawal signs
– determine the need for medication to relieve symptoms of nausea and vomiting; convulsion and delirium tremens	– to maintain physiological homeostasis – to minimize withdrawal symptoms – to decrease physical discomfort and physical complications
– provide comfort measures and emotional support during detoxification or withdrawal	– to provide reassurance that the experience is substance-related; to allay the fear and apprehension – panic reactions are not uncommon during detoxification – to maintain personal hygiene due to excessive perspiration, nausea and vomiting – to convey acceptance and interest
– provide high caloric diet and increase fluid intake	– to maintain hydration, replace fluid loss and re-establish nutritional deficiency – clients with substance disorders are often malnourished due to negligence and preference for use of substance rather than nutritional food
– health teach re: use of substance, tension-reducing techniques, side effects of use of combination substance, diet and rest	– most substance users use combination of drug and alcohol and are unaware of the drug interactions – to discuss with client some ways of substituting substance with other kind of beverages to lessen the addictive effects – to increase awareness of the long term effect of substance on overall functioning – to assist client develop other methods of coping with stress instead of substance abuse and dependence

Strategies	Rationale
Self-Concept Mode – see section on Anxiety, Chapter V and The Depressed Client, Chapter VII to:	
– observe for signs of anxiety, depression and suicidal attempts	– same
– assist with personal hygiene	– poor hygiene is not uncommon on clients with substance disorders – to provide opportunity for client to assist in self care and enhance self-esteem – to provide comfort measures and maintain good hygiene during the detoxification
– provide safe environment – see section on The Hyperactive Client,	– same – to provide quiet and safe environment while under the influence of substance – to provide safety precautions during the withdrawal or detoxification
– orientate to reality See section on The Withdrawn Client, Chapter VIII	– same – hallucination may occur during detoxification – to reassure client that the experience is drug related and will disappear shortly – to maintain contact with reality while under the influence of substance
– See section on The Aggressive Anti-Social Client, Chapter XI to:	
– assist client to express feelings	– same – to assess the pattern of substance abuse, i.e. type of substance used, frequency and amount
– display non-judgemental attitude	– threats may trigger panic reactions due to client's vulnerability – self doubt and low self-esteem are dominant and any notion of rejection will reinforce these feelings
Role Function Mode See section of The Aggressive Client, Chapter XI to:	
– set limits on behavior	– same
– be consistent on approach	– same
– assist client develop appropriate problem solving skills	– same

Strategies	Rationale
– engage client in constructive activities	– same
	– to test client's readiness for rehabilitation and type of therapy
	– to provide opportunities for education re substance abuse, work-related experiences
	– to motivate client in rehabilitation programs
	– to prepare client for rehabilitation and discharge planning
Interdependence Mode See section on The Aggressive Antisocial Client, Chapter XI to:	
– assist client to establish control of acting out behavior	– same
– teach client to regain control over sexual impulses	– same
– use confrontation appropriately	– same
– be aware of client's manipulative behavior	– same
– restrict visitors	– to prevent uncontrolled access to substance
– discuss with client and family treatment plan	– to involve family in client's rehabilitation program
	– to re-structure home activities satisfactorily without the use of any substance
	– to assist family deal with maladaptive behaviors displayed by client
	– to provide opportunities for family members to discuss their feelings and reactions
	– to promote consistency and continuity of treatment plan
	– family involvement is crucial to the effectiveness of rehabilitation
– assist client develop new social network and support system	– to foster peer support and pressure to develop behavior that is free of substance abuse
	– to prevent alienation and isolation
	– to enhance self-respect
	– to re-establish acceptance from others and lead a useful life
– provide information and referral regarding community health centres for follow-up care	– to ensure follow-up services as client usually drops out of clinics during bingeing episodes
	– to promote consistency and continuity of rehabilitation programs
	– to assist client and family become aware and make use of community self-help groups
	– immediate assistance should be available in the event that client needs help thus avoiding the use of any substance

EVALUATION

1. Assess the effectiveness of nursing actions and treatment plan.

2. Identify the factors that facilitated or hindered the plan of treatment.

3. Analyze your own reactions and attitudes toward clients with substance disorders.

Suggested Readings

Burgess, A. W., *Psychiatric Nursing in the Hospital and Community*. 3rd ed., Englewood Cliffs. Prentice Hall Publishing Co., 1981

Davis, C. & Schmidt, M., *Differential Treatment of Drug and Alcohol Abusers*. Palm Springs. ETC Publication, 1977

Glasser, F. et. al., *A System Approach to Alcohol Treatment*. Toronto. Addiction Research Foundation, 1978

Kolb, L. C., *Modern Clinical Psychiatry*. 10th ed., Philadelphia. W. B. Saunders Co., 1982

Wilson, H. & Kneisl, C., *Psychiatric Nursing*. 2nd ed., Menlo Park, California. Addison Wesley Publishing Co., 1983

Exercise 40

THE CLIENT WITH SUBSTANCE USE DISORDERS

Duration: 15 minutes

Direction: Answer the following questions. Think about it or discuss the topic in class.

1. Recall a person that you know, who is a substance user. What are the chief characteristics of his or her personality?

2. Describe the person's physical, emotional and mental state while under the influence of any of the substance.

3. Identify conditions that are likely to contribute to the use of the substance.

4. What would it be like to be this person's significant other, employer, subordinate, co-worker or friend?

5. As a nurse and friend of the family, list some specific nursing interventions that you will employ to assist the person and family.

CHAPTER 13

The Client with Serious Eating Disorders

In the last two decades there has been a shift in the attitude toward a thinner ideal female shape and that being slim is beautiful, desirable and admirable while being fat is utterly disgusting and unacceptable. This notion is exemplified by the proliferation of fashion and diet magazines, advertisements for weight clinics, diet ads, diet pills, gymnastic programs and so forth, all promising to take off the excess body weight.

By definition, anorexia means loss of appetite and anorexia nervosa is a severe weight loss due to self-imposed dietary restrictions to the point of starvation, commonly seen in young or adolescent females.

While anorexia means loss of appetite, anorexic usually experiences tremendous hunger and is preoccupied with food and eating. However, she denies herself food because of a growing sense that controlling food intake will increase her competencies and effectiveness as a person.

The decision to lose a few pounds often starts innocently with great satisfaction of being able to lose weight. Soon the anorexic realizes that her figure and appetite are the first things in her life that she can exercise some control. Coupled with the dieting, is the strenuous exercises and any attempt to moderate eating and exercise are met with extreme guilt.

Hence, preoccupation with food and calorie intake are meticulously accounted to, anxiously monitoring weight and daily progress. Once the desired weight loss is attained, the anorexic continues to diet ignoring the insistance of others to gain some weight. Consequently, she becomes extremely terrified of gaining some pounds, fearful of losing the new-found sense of control that her weight has produced.

In sum, if this condition occurs to someone who is vulnerable to anorexia nervosa, the condition may become a full blown disorder. Preoccupation with body fat that leads to such extreme behaviors such as vomiting after eating and use of laxatives indicate the need for immediate professional help.

THEORIES

Recent studies contradict the psychoanalytic theories of anorexia nervosa although some authorities still cannot ignore the existence of some deep seated emotional problems associated with unresolved oedipus complex, disturbed maternal-daughter relationship and family conflicts.

Anorexia nervosa is actually a disorder with multiple causation and each client has to be assessed on an individual basis. For some, the cause is related to an extreme need for self control that the client experiences from restriction of diet. Through control of food and their bodies, they feel that they have achieved control of their lives.

Another cause is related to feelings of inadequacies to meet the ever changing and increasing demands of growing up into adulthood. Sexual conflicts and fear of impregnation are often found at the base of this condition as one contemplates issues of dating, sex and marriage. Vocational decision and preparation for emancipation from a protective environment of home life, thin-slim conscious culture and the physical and physiological changes all add stress to the already existing feelings of apprehension and inadequacy.

The personality pattern of the client as a child was often found to be compliant, hypersensitive and avoided criticism, perfectionist and quite self-critical despite excellent performance and there is usually a close relationship with one or both parents. Parents of client are known to be weight and appearance conscious, athletic, place high demands and expectations for achievement on their children, overprotective, over-involved to the point of smothering the child.

ASSESSMENT
THE CLIENT WITH SERIOUS EATING DISORDERS

Physiological Mode	Self-Concept Mode	Role Function Mode	Interdependence Mode
– loss of weight (approximately 15% of the original body weight) – excessive dieting – food pre-occupation – poor concentration – decreased temperature, pulse, respiration, heart rate – dehydration – hair loss, lanugo at the back and face – dry skin – disturbed sleep pattern – constipation – self-induced vomiting – binge eating – menstrual cessation – absence of secondary sex characteristics – physical complaints, i.e. headaches, dizziness	– excessive concern with appearance, weight, bodily distortion, self-image – guilt, ambivalence – hypersensitivity to comments and criticisms – denial of illness and problems – perfectionist, self-critical – low self-esteem, inadequacy – manipulative, acting out behaviors – anxiety – withdrawal – depression	– compliant or negativistic – critical of self and others – controlling and manipulative – labile mood – tend to be perfectionist in role function – place high demands on expectations – able to form satisfactory interpersonal relation although on superficial level	– isolation – hypersensitive to comments of others – withdrawal – usually dissatisfied with life in general prior to onset of condition

PLANNING AND IMPLEMENTATION

Strategies	Rationale
Physiological Mode – check vital signs and observe physical condition of client	– to monitor bodily functions which are decreased due to starvation and to conserve energy. Overall metabolism is low so that fewer calories are required for survival – to prevent further weight loss – to determine the need for medication – to assess presence of other medical complications
– provide increased nutritional and caloric intake	– to re-establish hydration and nutritional intake – to promote weight gain – to re-establish electrolyte imbalance caused by starvation – to maintain adequate elimination
– maintain consistency of treatment approach	– to set and maintain strict limits regarding mealtime, amount of food intake, weighing and privileges – client tends to be manipulative, immature, especially during mealtime to take focus off eating

Strategies	Rationale
– set time limit and supervise mealtime	– to provide structure during mealtime as client tends to take her time in eating, attempts to hide food, hoards food and engorges self at a later time, attempts to manipulate staff members by acting out, crying, and so forth during meals
	– to determine the need for naso-gastric feeding if necessary
	– to check tray prior to meals for correct choice of menu. Client is most apt to choose low calorie food
	– to decrease association between food and stress
	– to ensure that client will eat the prescribed diet as she often leaves food untouched
	– to prevent binge eating
– supervise bathroom privileges after mealtime	– to prevent disposal of food, induce vomiting and concealment of weight gain
– set limits on physical and personal activities	– to conserve weight gain and disrupt further attempt to lose weight by strenuous exercise especially after meals
	– to prevent excessive bathing due to poor dry condition of the skin
Self-Concept Mode – assist client to express feelings	– to assess stress factors prior to weight loss; client's responses to stress
	– to assist client develop alternate methods rather than food-related coping mechanisms
	– to explore client's strengths and potential and build on these to increase self-esteem
	– to convey non-judgemental attitude and interest
Role Function Mode – decrease anger at staff members	– close supervision at mealtime and other activities is perceived as loss of control and autonomy
	– to provide opportunity for social interaction
	– to divert attention from food preoccupation
	– to increase social skills and problem solving skills
	– to decrease preoccupation with self-image
	– to maintain an optimum level of functioning
Interdependence Mode – decrease privileges until weight is gained	– to assist client establish satisfactory routine of eating habits and nutritional intake
	– to decrease environmental outside stressors until weight is gained
– involve family in treatment plan	– to promote continuity and consistency in rehabilitation
	– to facilitate positive interaction between family members and assist when necessary
	– family involvement is crucial to the effectiveness of treatment especially if there are family conflicts present

EVALUATION

1. Assess effectiveness of nursing intervention and treatment plan.

2. Identify the factors that influence or hinder the plan of care.

3. Suggest other methods of nursing actions.

Suggested Readings

Brush, H., *Eating Disorders: Anorexia Nervosa and the Person Within.* New York. Basic Books Inc., 1973

————. *The Golden Cage: The Enigma of Anorexia.* New York. Vintage Books, 1978

Erickson, E., *Identity: Youth and Crisis.* New York: W. W. Norton & Co., 1968

Haber, J. et al., *Comprehensive Psychiatric Nursing.* 2nd ed., New York. McGraw Hill Book Co., A Blakiston Publication, 1982

Jersild, A. T., *The Psychology of Adolescence.* 2nd ed., New York. MacMillan Co., 1963.

Lambert, V. & Lambert, C. E., *The Impact of Physical Illness and Related Mental Health Concepts.* Englewood Cliffs. Prentice Hall Publishing Co., 1979

Wilson, H. & Kneisl, C., *Psychiatric Nursing.* 2nd ed., Menlo Park, California. Addison Wesley Publishing Co., 1983

CHAPTER 14

The Confused-Disoriented Client

The increasing longevity and shift in the age make-up of the present population has given rise to a great many physiological, psychological, sociological and health problems which are now receiving more attention than ever before. It is speculated by leading authorities that some associated problems would be an increase in mental disorders of the aging population and the crucial problem becomes that of distinguishing normal changes with age and the pathological problems.

There are also a great number of other conditions which affect the central nervous system that may occur at any age giving rise to behavioral disturbances and dysfunctions. The clinical manifestation of a client with organic brain disorders will vary from person to person, may be displayed in a variety of functions and may range from mild to severe disturbances.

Organic brain disorders is defined as a disorder of physiological, psychological and behavioral functions caused by a damage to brain tissue. It is characterized by definite structural changes in the brain which is irreversible, for example, senility and pre-senile dementia such as Alzheimer's, Pick's, Huntington's, Korsakoffs' diseases and the like, the pre-senile conditions being commonly found in middle age. Organic brain disorders, however, is not always a part of the aging process.

Organic brain syndrome, on the other hand, are manifested by the symptomatology of organic brain disorders but are usually associated with other types of disorders. It may be transient or permanent, for example, head injuries, infections, endocrine dysfunctions, nutritional deficiencies, substance abuse and so forth. The degenerative effects of these disorders include a combination of both brain impairments and psychosocial deterioration.

The following conditions are potential causes of organic mental disorders.

1. Degenerative diseases such as Alzheimer, Pick, Huntington
2. Endocrine dysfunctions such as thyroid, parathyroid, adrenal
3. Metabolic and electrolyte imbalance
4. Vascular disorders such as hypertension, cerebral vascular accidents, congestive heart failures
5. Neoplastic disorders such as brain tumor, metastatic cancer
6. Infections such as CNS syphyllis, brain abcess, septicemia, meningoencephalitis, pneumonia
7. Nutritional deficiencies such as pernicious anemia, vitamin deficiencies especially thiamin, niacin, vitamin B–12, and iron deficiency
8. Substance abuse such as drug and alcohol
9. Toxic conditions such as heavy metals, solvents
10. Post traumatic reactions such as subdural hematoma, contusion
11. Epilepsy

THEORIES

Leading authorities believe that reactions of client toward organic brain disorders and organic brain syndromes are not only determined by the extent of neural damage but are also influenced by other variables such as the personality type and the kind of environment in which the client will continue to function. The growing awareness that psychosocial factors are far more significant to the optimum level of functioning has led to the consideration of the following.

A. Biological Aging

Biological aging brings degenerative processes that are characterized by decline in perceptual acuity, physical strength and coordination, capacity for learning, problem solving skills, ability to withstand stress, changes in appearance and increased vulnerability to illness. The vascular and nervous system are among the first to deteriorate and are commonly reflected in the reduction of psychomotor activities and increased intellectual rigidity. However, for those who have led an intellectually active life, there is minimum loss of intellectual functions and the client may continue to advance in life without significant changes, remain vigorous, productive and intellectually alert. Since the nervous system is the essential basis for integration of behavior, the extent of brain deterioration will determine the degree of impairment and will basically shape the pathology and character of disturbances, for example, the senility and presenile dementias.

B. Personality

Biological and psychological aging may either be hastened or retarded depending on the previous personality of the client and the life stresses that he or she has experienced. The severity of mental disorder will be influenced by the degree of previous intellectual functioning, emotional maturity and stability. Thus, the coping mechanism of the client prior to onset of illness will likely be the obvious maladaptive responses during the organic brain disorders. This stems from the fact that the brain damage limits the capacity to control the previous habits and attitudes. Deprived of the inhibition process, personality dispositions come to the surface in an unmodulated form and the client will likely exhibit marked accentuation of his or her personality traits in response to stress or release a latent personality disorder. For example, if the previous coping mechanism of the client to stressful events is to become depressed, withdrawn, suspicious, anxious, impulsive and so on, he or she will display most likely the same reactions. Similarly, a client who had favorable outlook in life and coped effectively with stress before illness will have imperceptible and minimal maladaptive behavior.

C. Sociological Factors

Together with biological and psychological aging is also what is commonly referred to as sociological aging. This notion reflects the changes in role function, position of the client in the family, the social role as well as societies attitude and expectation toward aging and mental illness. The realities of failing health, loss of status, becoming a burden to family intensifies the already existing feelings of fear and indignity of aging and add to the prospect of increased loneliness, poverty and social alienation.

Studies have shown that clients who are loved, cared for, and generally accepted, supported and encouraged by both family and society can withstand stress much better despite severe brain damage, with astonishing minimal brain disturbances and better prognosis. Conversely, a client who perceives hospitalization as a relief from life's worry and stress usually develop psychosis even in the presence of mild brain damage.

D. Dynamics of Behavior

Closely related to the personality of the client, it has been stated that the relation of organic conditions have minimal significance to the formation of maladaptive behaviors. Rather, these behaviors are more or less utilized as compensatory adaptation, albeit maladaptive, to reflect feelings of worthlessness, hopelessness, isolation and anxiety. The behaviors manifested are often displayed to manipulate the environment in order to establish some sense of order and meaning, to test reality. Thus, it enables the client to function in his or her old ways in spite of the structure limitation of the disorder. It may also take the form of grandiosity, withdrawal from tasks that deplete their limited capacities, rigidity in behavior and perseveration in the few things that he or she feel competent and comfortable. All these behaviors are protective mechanisms to compensate for the lowered or decreased capabilities and low self-esteem.

From biological point of view, although the regenerative capabilities of the central nervous system are limited and result in permanent destruction of the area affected, other parts of the system take over so that functions that are lost may be compensated for through re-learning. The degree of improvement may be limited or relatively complete, rapid or progressive or it may lead to permanent loss of function in cases of severe brain damage.

ASSESSMENT
THE CONFUSED DISORIENTED CLIENT

Physiological Mode	Self-Concept Mode	Role Function Mode	Interdependence Mode
Delirium (acute brain syndrome) – disorientation and disordered memory – confusion and distractibility – perceptual disturbance i.e. hallucination, illusion – increased or decreased psychomotor activities – sleep disturbances – speech disturbance, i.e. rambling, incoherent *Dementia* – progressive memory impairment, especially for recent events – deterioration of intellectual abilities – poor judgement, delusion, confabulation, echolalia – no clouding of consciousness – perseveration – personality changes – loss of sexual impulse control *Seizures and Convulsion* – petit mal – gran mal *Amnestic Syndrome* – short term memory loss without evidence of delirium and dementia *Bodily Emaciation* – vegetable like existence – bed ridden	– poor hygiene – labile shallow mood, i.e. laughter and tears without provocation – impulsive, irritability – marked apathy, indifference – hopelessness, worthlessness – loss of identity – withdrawal – suspicious – anxiety, agitation – pre-occupation with bodily functions, i.e. eating, digestion, excretion – no insight – decreased moral and ethical values	– grandiosity – lack of or decreased problem-solving skills – low tolerance for stress – unable to function independently – need assistance to perform activities of daily living – require time for completion of tasks – disrupted interpersonal relation – loss of status	– social detachment – withdrawal – mistrust others – impulsive – aggressive – negativistic – sexual acting out – fluctuation in interpersonal relation – loneliness – absence of significant others

Strategies	Rationale
Physiological Mode – monitor and increase nutritional food and fluid intake	– to maintain nutrition and hydration – to replace vitamin deficiencies – to ensure food and fluid intake as client may need assistance in feeding – to allay anxiety due to client's pre-occupation with bodily function – to promote quite, pleasant environment during mealtime as client is easily distracted – to avoid use of alcoholic beverages
– monitor elimination pattern	– to alleviate client's excessive concern with excretory function – inactivity, decrease roughage intake in diet, ingestion of drugs may cause constipation
– promote rest and sleep	– to re-establish healthy pattern of sleep and rest as client tends to wander around, confused, and disoriented during the night – client becomes easily irritated over slight noises and sudden movements that it interferes with rest and sleep – client becomes more fearful and apprehensive during the night; delirium and after convulsion – to provide an environment that is similar as closely as possible to usual surroundings thus to reduce disorientation
– provide safety measures	– to maintain necessary body equilibrium due to gross motor incoordination, i.e. sudden loss of balance, tendency to shift to one side when walking, jerky movements – to provide measures of control during delirium and convulsive seizures due to altered level of consciousness, hallucination, hyperactivity and sudden outburst of emotions – client easily responds to environmental stimuli and becomes excitable – client may not be able to perceive and understand signs of danger due to defective judgement – to anticipate an oncoming seizure and remove objects from mouth or other physical hazards – to reduce anxiety caused by cognitive disturbance
– orientate to reality See section on The Withdrawn Client, Chapter VIII	– same – presence of delirium may precipitate hallucination, disorientation and confusion – to re-establish identity and dignity brought by loss of memory, poor concentration, disorientation for time, place, events and people
– assess accurately physiological functions	– to prevent further illness, reserve energy and preserve present health as client is vulnerable to infections and other medical illness especially if bed-ridden – some clients may not experience pain and discomfort in conjunction with neurological impairment – in contrast, other clients will experience somatic complaints related to a particular illness – to assess effectiveness of drug therapy

173

Strategies	Rationale
Self-Concept Mode – assist with personal hygiene	– to ensure personal grooming and promote increased self-esteem – to re-establish self identity – client is usually not aware of the necessity of grooming due to forgetfulness, short attention span and worthlessness – gross motor incoordination often contribute to slovenly appearance – clients experiencing delirium and convulsive seizures will require immediate attention to hygiene after the acute episodes – immobility due to CVA will require assistance
– provide enough time for client to express self	– to re-establish self esteem if able to express self – client has difficulty communicating due to presence of aphasia, i.e. CVA – to facilitate expression as client is unable to express self spontaneously due to part of the brain affected, poor concentration span and memory loss – due to labile mood, feelings are expressed in accentuated form – to provide opportunity to assess client's thinking process and emotional responses
– provide safe environment	– to provide an atmosphere of acceptance and security in the event of acting out; delirium and convulsive seizures – client tends to get lost and wander due to confusion and disorientation – to provide close observation of clients' activities
– observe for signs of depression See Section on The Depressed Client, Chapter VII	– same – depression is frequently seen in organic brain disorders – the depressive reaction may be associated with previous personality make up
– observe factors that precipitate aggression. See section on The Aggressive Antisocial Client, Chapter XI	– same – client tends to be easily distracted and irritated. Acting out behaviors are common responses to frustration
Role Function Mode – engage and assist with familiar simple diversional activities	– to promote capacity for self renewal – to facilitate active interest in surroundings – to lessen anxiety in participation if activities are familiar due to difficulty in learning new things and rigidity in thinking and performance – to prevent further regression
– assist with daily activities of living	– to promote sense of success – poor concentration and short attention span makes the tasks difficult to accomplish – client is not able to perceive what he or she can do, hence direct supervision is required

Strategies	Rationale
– assist with problem solving skills if possible	– to utilize present potential skills and prevent further regression – to provide positive feedback and restore sense of dignity
Interdependence Mode – provide control of acting out behavior	– to provide security for the client and others – fluctuation of mood may lead to sudden acting out behavior – to protect client from self and others – to prevent rejection and further isolation from others
– provide control over sexual acting out	– to prevent discomfort created by sexual behavior in others – provide privacy for the client to meet sexual needs – to convey acceptance and non-judgemental attitude toward loss of control of sexual impulses
– involve family in treatment plan	– to convey an attitude of hopefulness – to prevent social detachment – family involvement is crucial to client's prognosis and to prevent further psychosocial deterioration – to provide opportunity for the family to express their concerns – to health teach the family re appropriate approach to client and the drug therapy in preparation for discharge

EVALUATION

1. Assess the effectiveness of nursing interventions and treatment plan.

2. Propose alternative nursing approaches if nursing actions are ineffective.

3. Analyze your own attitude toward aging process, specifically those clients with associated organic brain disorders.

Suggested Readings

Freedmen, A. M. et. al., *Comprehensive Textbook of Psychiatry II,* 2nd ed., Baltimore, Williams and Wilkins, 1979

Haber, J., et. al., *Comprehensive Psychiatric Nursing,* 2nd ed. New York. McGraw Hill Book Co., A Blakiston Publications, 1982

Kolb, L. C., *Modern Clinical Psychiatry,* 10th ed., Philadelphia. W. B. Saunders Co., 1982

Kyes, J. & Hofling, C., *Basic Psychiatric Nursing Concepts in Nursing,* 4th ed., Philadelphia. J. B. Lippincott Co., 1980

Peterson, C. G., *Organic Brain Syndrome.* Psychiatric Clinic of North America, Vol. 1, No. 1, April 1978

Stuart, G. W. and Sundeen, J. S., *Principles and Practice of Psychiatric Nursing,* 2nd ed. St. Louis. C. V. Mosby Co., 1983

Taylor, C. M., *Mereness' Essentials of Psychiatric Nursing,* 11th ed., St. Louis. The C. V. Mosby Co., 1982

Wilson, H. & Kneisl, C., *Psychiatric Nursing.* 2nd ed., Menlo Park, California. Addison Wesley Publishing Co., 1983

Exercise 41

THE CONFUSED-DISORIENTED CLIENT

Bill, an elderly male client, 55 years of age, was picked up by the police in the suburb of a large city, appearing dazed, cannot give his current address, somewhat restless and fidgety, his speech was slurred and the gait unsteady.

Upon admission to a psychiatric unit of a general hospital, the client was cooperative and pleasant but continuously mumbled to himself and displayed difficulty giving information. A few days after admission, Bill became quarrelsome and accused other clients of stealing his food. He was often found wandering aimlessly around the hospital grounds in his pajamas. During his short lucid moments, he was able to give the name of a relative who was then contacted by the hospital personnel.

According to his niece, Bill was a former police officer, a widower with no children and had just moved to Toronto from Vancouver after the death of his wife three years ago. Bill apparently has led quite an active life, has travelled extensively and both he and his wife had frequent bouts of drinking episodes during their married life. Since his transfer to Toronto, the niece noted some changes in his personality, refused to look for a job, lost interest in himself and others, and was frequently seen by the niece under the influence of alcohol. During his hospital stay, Bill would sit quietly and reminisce about his past life as a police officer and would frequently wait for his wife to visit. On occasions, he was able to give a detailed account of his activities but cannot remember whether he had his meals for the day or not. He often refused to participate in ward activities and states "I have to go to work, I don't have time now". Bill required assistance with his personal hygiene which was often neglected by the client.

1. Assess Bill's behavior according to:
   a. physiological mode

   b. self-concept mode

   c. role function mode

   d. interdependence mode

2. State your nursing diagnosis and formulate a plan of care for Bill.

3. Describe some of Bill's behavior that will reflect the following:
   a. dementia

   b. amnestic syndrome

   c. regression

   d. denial

   e. suspiciousness

   f. aggression

   g. lucid period

   h. confusion

   i. disorientation

4. What are the possible causes of Bill's condition?

5. List and describe the treatment modalities that will be likely prescribed for Bill.

6. What are the nursing problems that you might encounter during your nurse-client interaction with Bill? Why?

Exercise 42

MALADAPTIVE BEHAVIOR V

Duration: 10 minutes

Direction: State the diagnostic possibilities on the left hand blank space that you will anticipate for the following conditions.

_____ 1. Sheila has been highly febrile for the last few days, is restless and incoherent, agitated with alternating periods of drowsiness for short periods of time.

_____ 2. Joan spends a lot of time at a bar and frequently states that the wall paper was populated with pink elephants.

_____ 3. Irene, a 50 year old teacher, tells you that she went to a movie last night. A few minutes later, she tells you the same story all over again. This occurs many times during the day, together with carelessness in action and appearance.

_____ 4. Zeny has been suffering from severe headaches and has been told she has a brain tumor.

_____ 5. Bert, a 55 year old male, has unsteady gait, cannot speak coherently, often cries without tears, has poor concentration and becomes aggressive on occasion.

_____ 6. Paul is refused to participate in school sports due to frequent falls he takes whenever he has seizures.

_____ 7. Frederick fell and hit his head while playing hockey. Since then, he has been experiencing memory lapses.

_____ 8. Olga has been suffering from dizziness, headaches and occasional confusion especially after mixing the solution that she uses for cleaning floors every day at school where she works.

_____ 9. Perla is 70 years old and has managed her own business quite successfully until now when she begins to manifest labile mood, forgetfulness, hoarding of her belongings and some confusion.

_____ 10. Ann, who is now 83 years old, also has diabetis and hypertension. Recently, she displayed uncoordinated movements, gradual memory loss, difficulty remembering recent events and becomes disoriented as to time and place.

CHAPTER 15

Selected Treatment Modalities

This chapter focuses very briefly on the historical perspectives of treatment in psychiatry and outlines some of the current treatment approaches to provide familiarity with diversity of therapeutic interventions and beginning understanding of its rationale, goals and techniques.

The early recorded history suggest that mental illness has been co-existent with life and although there were no sophisticated diagnostic procedures and appraisal of mental disturbances at the time, it is reasonable to assume that some form of treatment existed.

In the past, disturbed client was thought to be possessed by an evil force and that relief can be obtained by efforts to drive out the evil which was present or to ease its exit from the body. Thus, holes were bored into the skull of the possessed so as to relieve pressure and permit the exit of the evil spirit.

Whipping and scourging were inflicted on the client but directed at the supernatural powers which was thought to be within the body and to cleanse the person of its possession. From this notion there evolved gradually the role of witch doctors, priest-physicians, exorcism, hypnotism and various group rituals to protect the community from invasion of the supernatural powers.

With increasing awareness of various behaviors, man began to relate his existence to the regularities of the world around him such as the lunar cycle, different seasons and other periodic occurrences and he began to recognize that his bodily ills were an expression of natural forces rather than supernatural powers. Part of the discovery was the realization that mental disturbances come from within rather than the effects of evil forces. When mental illness was perceived as consequence of natural phenomenon and not an expression of supernatural power or evil forces, scourging and other violent treatment, although still administered, was applied in an atmosphere of sympathy with attention given to physical hygiene. Thus, the recognition of humane approach in a calm and accepting environment, some form of massage and exercise, though still coupled with fear and apprehension on the part of the care giver, reduced the disturbed behavior drastically.

While the natural phenomenon concept was well underway, the relationship of the mind with physical functions began to gain some attention that led to the initial appreciation and recognition of the psychological origins of physiological disorders.

Ancient physicians of Greece have recorded the use of ataractic drugs, severe stimulations or psychological shocks in the form of immersion, cold or hot packs, or surprise baths. Counterpart treatments of music therapy, recreational and milieu therapies have also been recorded. Physical treatment was quite common and the use of psychological counselling has been largely confined to social class membership while other treatments mentioned previously were utilized mostly for lower socioeconomic class.

Although the nineteenth century brought new discoveries to the causation of mental illness and treatment approaches, the techniques utilized would only suggest that time has brought briefly refinement of treatment rather than innovations.

The healing touch of the Middle Age was replaced with healing words, physical symptoms were seen to respond favourably to counselling, the power of mind over body to produce and alleviate distress was revealed, the life history of the client and his learned patterns of adaption to account for his symptoms were acknowledged, and finally the discoveries of Freud.

With increased medical research there is recognition that gross pathological destruction or disruption of brain cells can produce behavioral disorders and that similar disorders can also be instigated by stress or other related factors in the absence of observable alteration in the structure and functions of the central nervous system.

In the early 1930's treatment of schizophrenia by intramuscular injection of camphor in oil postulated a biological antagonism between epilepsy and schizophrenia since epilepsy is rarely found in schizophrenics. Problems of control of seizures however, caused massive anxiety on clients and the convulsive seizures were found to be more effective to relieve signs and symptoms of melancholia. Manfred Sakel suggested in 1935 that hypoglycemic coma might alleviate the symptoms of schizophrenia and the hypothesis was based on his treatment of the withdrawal symptoms of morphine addicts by injection of insulin. Carlleti and Bini introduced the use of electric current across the frontal lobe of the brain to achieve a controlled epileptic seizure in 1937, now commonly known as electroconvulsive therapy (ECT).

The use of drugs during this time was on the basis of symptomatic treatments only due to absence of generally agreed upon rationale and limited experimentation and the drugs used had immediate effects on the central nervous system that put the client into coma.

Although medical treatment of mental illness became established and accepted as therapy of choice for specific disorders, these approaches continue to undergo significant changes. Despite the argument for the use of physical treatment to ameliorate symptomatology the client is generally treated with either physical treatment such as chemotherapy and electroconvulsive therapy or with intense therapeutic interactions.

Within psychiatry, there are psychiatrists who treat almost exclusively by administration of drugs, ECT or other physical means and on the other hand, there are psychiatrists who almost treat only by psychotherapy.

It is not uncommon, however, to note in many instances that medical and psychological models are jointly prescribed.

While the period of concentrated development of medical model occurred in the early thirties, the last two decades saw a progressive erosion of psychological approaches and discovery of new drugs that afforded a critical approach to treatment modalities.

Types of Treatment

A. *Electroconvulsive therapy*

The treatment consists of passing an electrical current by the use of a machine which cannot deliver an electrocution dose across the frontal lobe of the brain. The current is transmitted through the use of electrodes placed either bilaterally or unilaterally on the temporal areas of the skull and causes an electrical stimulation of the brain which produces a convulsion simliar to a Gran Mal epileptic seizure.

It is used to disrupt the client's ongoing patterns of thinking, feeling and behaving thus establishing new patterns of responses, making the client more accessible to others and hastening of psychotherapeutic process. Although the exact mechanism is still unknown, there is ample evidence of its biochemical responses and is found to be quite effective for major affective disorders. The psychological interpretation of the effects states that its action may also serve as a symbolic punishment for client who feels guilty and worthless. Another theory proposes that ECT is perceived as life-threatening experiences thereby mobilizing the bodily defenses to counteract the attack. The client may experience some confusion, memory loss and other somatic complaints especially headaches during the course of the treatment which usually ceases upon completion of the treatment.

B. *Chemotherapy*

The use of chemotherapy has come to occupy a major place in the treatment of mental illness and not only do the drugs alleviate the symptoms of the illness but also provide much wider scheme of rehabilitation and out-patient treatments. However, the great breakthrough with all its encouraging results has not been wthout any hazards and problems. Concomitant with the use of drugs are the dangers of addiction, overdosage, drug sensitivity and drug toxicity which produces undesirable long or permanent side effects.

Psychotropic agents are those drugs that are effective in the treatment of psychosis, major affective and anxiety disorders. It may be most conveniently classified as, namely:

1. Antipsychotic agents

   It is also known as major tranquillizers, ataractic or neuroleptic drugs and are most effective in the treatment of psychosis. They act on the chemical transmitters near the synaptic connections in the central nervous system. It selectively inhibits the chemoreceptor zone, the hypothalamus and the reticular formation thus interrupting the impulses coming through this area to the cortex and result in the depression of certain subcortical sites that are involved in the emotional reactivity of the client. Thus it promotes a state of calmness and relaxation with suppression of excessive emotional behavior.

   Phenothiazine derivatives are the most common examples of the group agents, for example, Haloperidol, Trifluoperazine, Chlorpromazine, Fluphenazine, and so forth.

2. Antidepressant agents

   Also known as psychic energizers due to their energy-producing and mood elevating actions which stimulated depressed clients to become more involved in themselves and their environment. The agents may be classified into tricyclic group and the monoamine oxidase inhibitors (MAO).

   The MAO inhibitor drugs inhibit the enzyme monoamine oxidase that destroy certain neurohormones such as epinephrine, norepinephrine, and serotonin which are responsible for stimulating the physical and mental activities. It is also believed that MAO inhibitors are responsible for maintaining an equilibrium within the body by increasing the life span of the neurohormones. The tricyclic drugs is hypothesized to affect brain amine levels by interfering with amine binding ability.

   The most common MAO inhibitors utilized are Isocarboxazid, Phenelzine and the tricyclic drugs are the Amitriptyline, Imipramine, Doxepin and the like.

3. Antianxiety agents

   These drugs are commonly known as minor or mild tranquilizers used to alleviate anxiety in anxiety and somatoform disorders. It acts by depressing the neurotransmitter to decrease the impact of stimulus reaction and response.

   The drug is also used for control of substance abuse withdrawal symptoms and in any other conditions in which agitation, tension and anxiety play a significant role. The drugs commonly used are Diazepam, Chlordiazepoxide, Meprobamate and so forth.

4. Antimanic agent

   The drug is commonly known as Lithium Carbonate and was first used in the early 70's to treat the manic and hypomanic phase of Bipolar disorders. Although many other overactive clients respond well to Lithium Carbonate, in others the response is not as effective and the drug can cause serious side effects, including interference with sodium level in the body. The mechanism of action is still not clearly understood but it is thought to block the release of norepinephrine and stimulate its uptake at the neural synapse. For clients with affective bipolar disorders, the drug may be used for prophylactic treatment to reduce the severity and frequency of the manic episodes.

5. Other drugs used in psychiatry

   The anticholinergic drugs such as Benztropine Mezylate and Trihexyphenidyl are commonly administered because of their property to control the induced extrapyramidal reactions often caused by antipsychotic drugs. The action is to block acetylcholine released by nerve endings at certain cerebral synaptic sites.

   For further information and current use of drugs the reader is referred to pharmacology textbooks or other drug compendium.

C. *Psychological Approach*

In the early origins of psychological management the Greek-Roman physicians were not without psychological impact although there were no explicit references to the term psychotherapy. Some elements of the present psychotherapeutic interventions were present in their approach to clients. For example, the client was perceived, treated and respected as an individual and involved time spent with the treatment specifically prescribed based on client's personal needs.

1. Psychotherapy

Psychotherapy is one of the earliest forms of psychological treatment and yet the latest treatment to achieve scientific recognition. The origin of modern psychotherapy is generally conceded to begin with Freud, the therapy and techniques to which he first applied the term psychoanalysis in 1896.

It is used in a variety of ways and in its broadest sense psychotherapy may be anything from a comforting word or supportive action to a prolonged intensive process. The methods and techniques cannot be standardized as the choice of intervention is determined by the needs of the client and therapist's competency and theoretical orientation.

However, as defined by the American Psychiatric Association Glossary, psychotherapy "is a process in which a person who wishes to change symptoms or problems in living or in seeking personal growth, enter, implicitly or explicitly, into a contract to interact in a prescribed way with a psychotherapist". The application of psychotherapy may either be individual or in a group, directive or non-directive.

Types of individual psychotherapy

a. Supportive psychotherapy

It is a directive approach to assist the client achieve ways of controlling impulses, seek relief from present problems or emotional upheaval and strengthen the present healthy coping skills through utilization of encouragement and giving reassurance, ventilation, clarifying the problem, persuasion and suggestion, direct teaching and manipulation of the environment. Probing into the unconscious past experiences is avoided and the focus is on the presenting problems.

b. Psychoanalysis

Originally developed by Freud, its goal is the uncovering and modification of unconscious psychological forces that occurred in childhood. It is a method of psychotherapy based on a body of facts and theories, linking the past with the present and associating the feelings with repressed conflicts. Its principles are based upon the principles of the unconscious content, free association, analysis of dream, transference and countertransference, interpretation and resistance.

The use of psychoanalysis nowadays seems to be limiting because of the length of time involved and large expenditure incurred. However, the insights gained from it have been significant and helpful in other forms of therapy and quite often characterize the process of most therapy.

c. Hypnotherapy

It is an artificially induced state of relaxation where a client becomes prone to suggestion or re-enacts deeper emotional experiences. It is utilized to facilitate psychotherapy and at times to eliminate maladaptive behaviors that a client may wish to give up but for some reason cannot.

d. Client Centered therapy

Introduced by Roger, the approach is based on humanistic philosophy and involves the use of empathic understanding and self exploration. Through permissive relationship with the therapist, the therapist reflects the client's feelings by using non-directive techniques and offers total acceptance. The client then gains positive regard for self that leads to self-actualization.

e. Gestalt therapy

The approach of Perls to the therapy although humanistic in nature is more technique oriented. It utilizes the applications of rules and games, re-enactment of conversation with one's own feelings or with other persons or objects for the purpose of catharsis. The aim of the therapy is to assist the client acknowledge the here and now feelings and its immediate resolution to prevent their avoidance in order to restore the person to a sense of wholeness.

2. Group Psychotherapy

The use of group process (Chapter 3) in psychiatry is more directed toward psychotherapeutic intervention. Although it is similar in its principles, the process is different based on the goals of the group, membership participation, size and structure of the group, length of contract and its sessions and the role of the trained therapist.

The techniques used in group therapy parallel those utilized in individual psychotherapy with the exception of its application to a number of six to eight clients in a given group setting. The group approach is often used in conjunction with individual psychotherapy.

There are also various group activities mentioned in Chapter 3 that are utilized in psychiatry that proved to have psychotherapeutic values and are commonly used as adjuncts to psychiatric treatments.

3. Behavior therapy

Behavior therapy in its broadest sense refers to all types of therapeutic interventions that are derived from principles of learning. It is a method of altering socially unacceptable behaviors on the basis of positive and negative reinforcement. The process of the therapy is based on the behavior to be altered, the environmental conditions that support the behavior and the changes to be made in the environment to correct the behavior.

The types of behavior therapy techniques most widely used are:

a. Desensitization

It is a technique developed by Wolpe which associates anxiety producing stimuli with a relaxation response to the stimuli. Hopefully, through repeated conditioning the increased relaxation responses will decrease the fear response to the same stimuli thus making the client free of the fear and acquire new adaptive responses.

b. Aversion therapy

Although closely related to desensitization, aversion technique seeks to eliminate undesirable behaviors. Based on the classical Pavlovian conditioning process the stimuli are associated with unpleasant strong responses. Desensitization, on the other hand, attempts to eliminate responses that inhibits desirable behaviors.

c. Implosive therapy

Again, it is a technique which is quite similar to desensitization in terms of its goals and procedure. It only differs in that the therapist seeks to frighten or flood the client with overwhelming stimulation in a setting in which no actual harm can occur. Consequently the client gradually learns that the fears are unfounded and eventually gives up the maladaptive responses.

d. Behavior modification

Based on the modification of responses through reward, the technique employed utilizes the "token economy" where appropriate changes in behaviors are rewarded with a token that a client can exchange for privileges, cigarettes, food, and the like.

e. Cognitive behavior therapy

It is a technique recommended by Beck for treatment of depression to correct the negative mental set of the client about himself or herself. The negative expectation that the client anticipates from the environment promotes and perpetuates his or her difficulties in life. It is a more active process and the strategy is to redirect the client's misguided attitude and focus more on functional thoughts and behavior. Assertive training techniques may be utilized to interfere and correct the faulty beliefs of the client and acquire new adaptive behavior and responses.

f. Rational Emotive therapy

The approach is formulated by Ellis whose goal is to change maladaptive behaviors which resulted from the client's illogical and irrational beliefs.

The client is induced to think and verbalize these negative beliefs, then attacks them and tells the client to engage in a mental set or activities using positive imagination which run parallel to the negative attitude. Through confrontation of the irrational beliefs, the client adapts a more rational attitude by which he or she can live with.

4. Milieu therapy

Based on sociocultural approach to treatment, the implementation of milieu therapy was stimulated by the work of Maxwell Jones in the early 1950's.

The approach is based on the concept of therapeutic community to assist the clients learn new adaptive behaviors. The unit is specifically designed to simulate the life and activities of the outside social world with major emphasis on teaching the client to behave in a socially acceptable manner, assuming of responsibility in the overall treatment plan through client government, practice open ward policies and enhance communication between staff members and client.

5. Family therapy

It is a form of group therapy based on the notion that the emotional disturbances of individual members of the family is regarded as an outgrowth of conflicts between family members, the client being merely its most dramatic symptom. The most common techniques of family therapy are those developed by Ackerman and Satir where all members of the family are brought together and areas of conflicts and communications were explored. The aim of the therapy is to dissolve the barriers to communication, to neutralize the negative feelings among the members and to explore healthier patterns of relating to one another.

D. *Crisis Intervention*

In the last few decades research and the influence of the 1961 Report of the Joint Commission on Mental Illness and Health in the United States, has produced new concepts called crisis theory and crisis intervention that have proved quite helpful and contributed significantly to mental health delivery services and in the development of community mental health movement.

These concepts stem from the notion that not only is everyone subject to stressful life events and life threatening situations but these changes have the potentials of becoming a crisis. That is, during certain stressful situations in life people are more susceptible to crises than during others. Human individuality will cause one person to bypass such a period whereas another person may be engulfed by it, rendering that person incapable of coping with the stress and the likelihood of crises.

Crisis does not necessarily follow a traumatic event, neither do the events of life activate crisis. Whether such predicaments and events become a crisis depends upon the ability of the individual to handle the stresses and the presence of support system.

Crisis may be described as a state of emotional disequilibrium characterized by increased inner tension and anxiety, disorganization of function and inability to solve problems in their usual way. According to Caplan, crisis is any situation that causes a sudden alteration in the individual's expectation of himself with others; it is a self limiting process that lasts from four to six weeks; it is a transition period that makes the person psychologically vulnerable; and that the crisis provides an opportunity for personal growth.

Allowing for differences in human beings and the nature of crises that may occur, crisis may be categorized as:

1. Maturational crisis—an event that describes the unique stresses that occur during the developmental phase of growth and development which begins from birth to death. Generally the individual experiences a higher level of anxiety while going through the transition changes in body image and functions, roles and ways of relating to self and outside world, than at other times. Recognition of these stresses in each of the developmental phase aids in preventing a potential crisis from becoming a full blown crisis.

2. Situational crises—are events that occur as a result of some unanticipated traumatic incident that is usually beyond one's control. Common situational events are: loss either by illness, death, separation, status and role change, and natural disaster.

Unlike maturational crisis, situational crisis is generally unforeseen and there is nothing that one can do to prepare for it. While one cannot predict the situational events that may precipitate crises, one can anticipate the pattern of reaction as a response to the event, i.e. stages of grief and grieving process.

Crisis intervention is a short term helping process which is not synonymous with psychotherapy even though some communication techniques may be used in both. Besides the technical aspect of communication techniques, crisis intervention involves anticipatory guidance, immediate restoration of the person to a pre-crisis state, provision of immediate support, search for alternate methods of coping and assessment of suicidal and homicidal risks.

The following table illustrates the differences between psychotherapy and crisis intervention.

	Psychotherapy	Crisis Intervention
Goals of therapy	- restructuring of personality - removal of specific symptoms	- resolution of crisis - development of other methods of coping - participatory support system
Focus of treatment	- genetic past as it relates to present - repression of unconscious drives	- restoration to level of function prior to crisis
Activity of therapist	- passive participant - non-directive approach - interpretive - explanatory	- active participant - direct approach - functional
Problem areas	- chronic, emotional illness	- sudden loss of ability to try to cope with life situation
Length of Treatment	- indefinite	- 1-6 sessions

Figure 15.1 Differences Between Psychotherapy and Crisis Intervention

Suggested Readings

Bellack, A. & Hersen, M., *Behavior Modification: An Introductory Textbook*. Baltimore. Williams and Wilkins, 1977
Beck, A., *The Development of Depression: A Cognitive Model, The Psychology of Depression*. Contemporary Theory and Research. Washington, D.C. V. H. Winston, 1974
Kolb, L. C., *Modern Clinical Psychiatry*. 10th ed., Philadelphia. W. B. Saunders Co., 1982
Kyes, J. & Hofling, C., *Basic Psychiatric Concepts in Nursing*. 4th ed., Philadelphia. J. B. Lippincott Co., 1980
Marram, G. D., *The Group Approach in Nursing Practice*. St. Louis. C. V. Mosby Co., 1973
Schaefer, H. & Martin, P., *Behavior Therapy*. 2nd ed., New York. McGraw Hill Book Co., 1975
Yalom, I., *The Theory and Practice of Group Psychotherapy*. New York. Basic Books Publishers, 1971

REFERENCES

American Psychiatric Association. *Diagnostic and Statistical Manual of Mental Disorders.* Washington, D.C. APA 1980

Aguilera, D. C., et. al., *Crisis Intervention:* Theory and Methodology. 2nd ed., St. Louis. C. V. Mosby Co., 1974

Aguilera, D. C. & Topalis, M., *Psychiatric Nursing.* 7th ed. St. Louis. The C. V. Mosby Co., 1978

Bandura, A., *Aggression: A Social Learning Analysis.* Englewood Cliffs. Prentice Hall, 1983

Beck, A., *The Development of Depression: A Cognitive Model, The Psychology of Depression.* Contemporary Theory and Research. Washington, D.C., V. H. Winston, 1974

Benne, J. D. & Sheates, P., *Functional Roles of Group Members.* J. Social Issues. 4:41–49, 1949

Bellack, A., Hersen, M., *Behavior Modification: An Introductory Textbook.* Baltimore. Williams and Wilkins, 1977

Birren, J. E. & Warner, S. K., *Handbook of the Psychology of Aging.* New York. Van Nostrand Reinholft Co., 1977

Blake, K. & Taylor, C. E., *The Prevention and Management of Aggressive Behavior.* Columbia, South Carolina Department of Mental Health, 1977

Blondis, M. N. & Jackson, E., *Non-Verbal Communication with Patients.* New York. A Wiley Medical Publication, 1977

Bonner, H., *Group Dynamics: Principle and Application.* New York. Ronald Press, 1964

Brush, H., *Eating Disorders: Anorexia Nervosa and the Person Within.* New York. Basic Books Inc., 1973

Burd, S. M. & Marshall, M. A., *Some Clinical Approaches to Psychiatric Nursing.* New York. MacMillan & Co., 1963

Burgess, A. W., *Psychiatric Nursing in the Hospital and Community.* 3rd ed., Englewood Cliffs. Prentice Hall Inc., 1981

————. *The Golden Cage: The Enigma of Anorexia.* New York. Vintage Books, 1978

Burnside, I. M., *Psychosocial Nursing Care of the Aged.* New York. McGraw Hill Book Co., 1973

Butler, R. & Lewis, M. I., *Aging and Mental Health.* St. Louis. The C. V. Mosby Co., 1978

Carkhuff, R., et. al., *The Art of Helping III.* Amherst, Mass. Human Resource Development Press, 1977

Carlson, C. E., *Behavioral Concepts and Nursing Interventions.* Philadelphia. J. B. Lippincott Publishing, 1979

Cartwright, D. & Zander, A., *Group Dynamics: Research and Theory.* New York. Harper & Row Publishers, 1968

Cattal, R. B. & Scheir, I. N., *Theory and Research on Anxiety: Anxiety Behavior.* New York. Academic Press, 1966

Chambers, C. C., *Nursing Concepts and Processes.* Albany, New York. Delmar Publishers, 1977

Chenevert, M., *Special Techniques in Assertive Training for Women in the Health Profession.* St. Louis. The C. V. Mosby Co., 1978

Clark, C. C., *The Nurse as a Group Leader.* New York. Springer Publishing Co., 1977

Collins, M., *Communication in Health Care.* 2nd ed. St. Louis. The C. V. Mosby Co., 1983

Coombs, A., et. al., *Helping Relationships.* 2nd ed. Boston, Mass. Allyn & Bacon Inc., 1978

Davis, C. & Schmidt, M., *Differential Treatment of Drug and Alcohol Abusers.* Palm Springs. ETC Publication, 1977

Dunlap, L. C., *Mental Health Concepts Applied to Nursing.* New York. A. Wiley Publications, 1978

Edwards, B. J. & Brilhart, K. C., *Communication in Nursing Practice.* St. Louis. The C. V. Mosby Co., 1981

Erickson, E., *Identity: Youth & Crisis.* New York. W. W. Norton and Co., 1968

Farberow, N. L., Shneidman eds., *The Cry For Help.* New York. McGraw Hill Book Co., 1961

Freud, S., *The Problem of Anxiety.* New York. Norton Press, 1963

Gerrad, B., et. al., *Interpersonal Skills for Health Professionals.* Reston, Virginia. Reston Publishing Co., Inc. A Prentice Hall Co., 1980

Glasser, P. & et. al., *A System Approach to Alcohol Treatment.* Toronto. Addiction Research Foundation, 1978

Haber, J. & et. al., *Comprehensive Psychiatric Nursing.* 2nd ed. New York. McGraw Hill Book Co., A Blakiston Publication, 1982

Hays, J. S. & Larsen, K. H., *Interacting with Patient.* New York. MacMillan Co., 1969

Hinsie, L. & Campbell, R., *Psychiatric Dictionary.* 4th ed. New York. Oxford University Press, 1970

Hoff, L. A., *People in Crisis—Understand and Helping.* Menlo Park, California. Addison Wesley Publishing Co., 1978

Jersild, A. T., *The Psychology of Adolescence.* 2nd ed. New York. MacMillan Co., 1963

Klein, J., *The Study of Groups.* The International Library of Sociology and Social Reconstruction. London. Routledge and Paul Ltd., 1965

Knowles, M. & Knowles, H., *Introduction to Group Dynamics.* New York. Association Press, 1959

Kolb, L. C., *Modern Clinical Psychiatry.* 10th ed. Philadelphia. W. B. Saunders Co., 1982

Kreigh, H. Z. & Perko, J. E., *Psychiatric Mental Health Nursing: Commitment of Care and Concern.* 2nd ed. Reston, Virginia. Reston Publishing Co., A Prentice Hall Co., 1983

Kyes, J. & Hofling, C., *Basic Psychiatric Concepts in Nursing.* 4th ed. Philadelphia. J. B. Lippincott Co., 1980

Lambert, V. & Lambert, C. E., *The Impact of Physical Illness and Related Mental Health Concepts.* Englewood Cliffs. Prentice Hall Inc., 1979

Lewton, K., *Field Theory in Social Service.* D. Cartwright, ed., New York. Harper & Brothers, 1951

Lewinsohn, P. M., et. al., *Sensitivity of Depressed Individuals to Aversive Stimuli.* Journal of Abnormal Psychology '81, pp 259–263, 1973

Marram, G. D., *The Group Approach in Nursing Practice.* St. Louis. The C. V. Mosby Co., 1977

Masserman, J. H., *Principles of Dynamic Psychiatry.* Philadelphia. W. B. Saunders, 1961

Millon, Theodore, *Disorders of Personality.* DSM III. Axis II. New York. John Wiley & Sons, 1981

Mitchell, P. H., *Concepts Basic to Nursing.* 2nd ed., New York. McGraw Hill Book Co., 1977

Noonan, K. A., *Emotional Adjustment to Illness.* Albany, New York. Delmar Publishers, 1975

Peplau, H. E., *A Working Definition of Anxiety in Some Clinical Approaches to Psychiatric Nursing*. New York. MacMillan Co., 1973

Poznanski, E. & Zrull, J. P., *Childhood Depression: Cinical Characteristic of Overtly Depressed Children*. Archives of General Psychiatry. 23, pp 8–15, 1970

Randall, E. & et. al. *Adaptation Nursing: The Roy Conceptual Model Applied*. St. Louis. The C. V. Mosby Co., 1982

Roberts, S., *Behavioral Concepts and Nursing Throughout the Life Span*. Englewood Cliffs. Prentice Hall Inc., 1978

Robinson, L., *Psychiatric Nursing As a Human Experience*. Philadelphia. W. B. Saunders Co., 1972

Roy, Sister C., *Introduction to Nursing: An Adaptation Model*. Englewood Cliffs, Prentice Hall Inc., 1976

Rutter, M., *Childhood Schizophrenia Reconsidered*. J. Autism. Childhood Schizophrenia. 2, 315–337, 1872

Schaefer, H. & Martin, P., *Behavior Therapy*. 2nd ed. New York. McGraw Hill Book Co., 1975

Schultz, J. & Dark, S., *Manual of Psychiatric Nursing Care Plans*. Boston. Little, Brown & Co., 1982

Selligman, M., *Depression and Learned Helplessness*. The Psychology of Depression, Contemporary Theory and Research. Washington, D.C. V. H. Winston, 1974

Spitz, R., *The Psychoanalytic Study of the Child*. New York. International University Press, 1965

Stegne, L., *The Prevention and Management of Disturbed Behavior*. Toronto. Ontario Government Book Store. 1977

Stuart, C. W. & Sundeen, S. J., *Principles and Practice of Psychiatric Nursing*. 2nd ed., St. Louis. The C. V. Mosby Co., 1983

Taylor, C. M., *Mereness' Essentials of Psychiatric Nursing*. 11th ed. St. Louis. The C. V. Mosby Co., 1982

Topalis, M., & Aguilera, D., *Psychiatric Nursing*. 7th ed. St. Louis. The C. V. Mosby Co., 1978

Whitaker, D. S., *A Group Centred Approach*. Group Process. 7:37–57, 1967

Wilson, H. & Kneisl, C., *Psychiatric Nursing*. 2nd ed. Menlo Park, California. Addison Wesley Publishing Co., 1983

Yalom, I., *The Theory and Practice of Group Psychotherapy*. New York. Basic Books Publishers, 1971

DSM-III Classification
Axis I-V

All official DSM-III codes and terms are included in ICD–9–CM. However, in order to differentiate those DSM-III categories that use the same ICD–9–CM codes, unofficial non-ICD–9–CM codes are provided in parentheses for use when greater specificity is necessary.

The long dashes indicate the need for a fifth-digit subtype or other qualifying term.

AXES I AND II: CATEGORIES AND CODES

Disorders Usually First Evident in Infancy, Childhood or Adolescence

Mental Retardation (Code in fifth digit: 1 = with other behavioral symptoms [requiring attention or treatment and that are not part of another disorder], 0 = without other behavioral symptoms.)

317.0(x)   Mild Mental Retardation, _____
318.0(x)   Moderate Mental Retardation, _____
318.1(x)   Severe Mental Retardation, _____
318.2(x)   Profound Mental Retardation, _____
319.0(x)   Unspecified Mental Retardation, _____

Attention Deficit Disorder

314.01   with Hyperactivity
314.00   without Hyperactivity
314.80   Residual Type

Conduct Disorder

312.00   Undersocialized, Aggressive
312.10   Undersocialized, Nonaggressive
312.23   Socialized, Aggressive
312.21   Socialized, Nonaggressive
312.90   Atypical

Anxiety Disorders of Childhood or Adolescence

309.21   Separation Anxiety Disorder
313.21   Avoidant Disorder of Childhood or Adolescence
313.00   Overanxious Disorder

Other Disorders of Infancy, Childhood, or Adolescence

313.89   Reactive Attachment Disorder of Infancy
313.22   Schizoid Disorder of Childhood or Adolescence
313.23   Elective Mutism
313.81   Oppositional Disorder
313.82   Identity Disorder

Eating Disorders

307.10   Anorexia Nervosa
307.51   Bulimia
307.52   Pica
307.53   Rumination Disorder of Infancy
307.50   Atypical Eating Disorder

Stereotyped Movement Disorders

307.21   Transient Tic Disorder
307.22   Chronic Motor Tic Disorder
307.23   Tourette's Disorder
307.20   Atypical Tic Disorder
307.30   Atypical Stereotyped Movement Disorder

Other Disorders with Physical Manifestations

307.00   Stuttering
307.60   Functional Enuresis
307.70   Functional Encopresis
307.46   Sleepwalking Disorder
307.46   Sleep Terror Disorder (307.49)

Pervasive Developmental Disorders Code in fifth digit: 0 = Full Syndrome Present, 1 = Residual State.

299.0x   Infantile Autism, _____
299.9x   Childhood Onset Pervasive Developmental Disorder, _____
299.8x   Atypical, _____

Specific developmental disorders
Note: These are coded on Axis II.

315.00   Developmental Reading Disorder
315.10   Developmental Arithmetic Disorder
315.31   Developmental Language Disorder
315.39   Developmental Articulation Disorder
315.50   Mixed Specific Developmental Disorder
315.90   Atypical Specific Developmental Disorder

Source: The American Psychiatric Association, Diagnostic and Statistical Manual of Mental Disorders, Third Edition, Washington, D.C., APA 1980. Reprinted by permission.

Organic Mental Disorders

Section 1. Organic Mental Disorders whose etiology or pathophysiological process is listed below (taken from the mental disorders section of ICD–9–CM).

Dementias Arising in the Senium and Presenium

Primary Degenerative Dementia, Senile Onset,
290.30 with Delirium
290.20 with Delusions
290.21 with Depression
290.00 Uncomplicated
Code in fifth digit:
1 = with Delirium, 2 = with Delusions, 3 = with Depression, 0 = Uncomplicated.
290.1x Primary Degenerative Dementia, Presenile Onset, _____

290.4x Multi-infarct Dementia, _____

Substance-induced

ALCOHOL
303.00 Intoxication
291.40 Idiosyncratic Intoxication
291.80 Withdrawal
291.00 Withdrawal Delirium
291.30 Hallucinosis
291.10 Amnestic Disorder
Code severity of Dementia in fifth digit: 1 = Mild, 2 = Moderate, 3 = Severe, 0 = Unspecified.
291.2x Dementia Associated with Alcoholism, _____

BARBITURATE OR SIMILARLY ACTING SEDATIVE OR HYPNOTIC
305.40 Intoxication (327.00)
292.00 Withdrawal (327.01)
292.00 Withdrawal Delirium (327.02)
292.83 Amnestic Disorder (327.04)

OPIOID
305.50 Intoxication (327.10)
292.00 Withdrawal (327.11)

COCAINE
305.60 Intoxication (327.20)

AMPHETAMINE OR SIMILARLY ACTING SYMPATHOMIMETIC
305.70 Intoxication (327.30)
292.81 Delirium (327.32)
292.11 Delusional Disorder (327.35)
292.00 Withdrawal (327.31)

PHENCYCLIDINE (PCP) OR SIMILARLY ACTING ARYLCYCLOHEXYLAMINE
305.90 Intoxication (327.40)
292.81 Delirium (327.42)
292.90 Mixed Organic Mental Disorder (327.49)

HALLUCINOGEN
305.30 Hallucinosis (327.56)
292.11 Delusional Disorder (327.55)
292.84 Affective Disorder (327.57)

CANNABIS
305.20 Intoxication (327.60)
292.11 Delusional Disorder (327.65)

TOBACCO
292.00 Withdrawal (327.71)

CAFFEINE
305.90 Intoxication (327.80)

OTHER OR UNSPECIFIED SUBSTANCE
305.90 Intoxication (327.90)
292.00 Withdrawal (327.91)
292.81 Delirium (327.92)
292.82 Dementia (327.93)
292.83 Amnestic Disorder (327.94)
292.11 Delusional Disorder (327.95)
292.12 Hallucinosis (327.96)
292.84 Affective Disorder (327.97)
292.89 Personality Disorder (327.98)
292.90 Atypical or Mixed Organic Mental Disorder (327.99)

Section 2. Organic Brain Syndromes whose etiology or pathophysiological process is either noted as an additional diagnosis from outside the mental disorders section of ICD–9–CM or is unknown.

293.00 Delirium
294.10 Dementia
294.00 Amnestic Syndrome
293.81 Organic Delusional Syndrome
293.82 Organic Hallucinosis
293.83 Organic Affective Syndrome
310.10 Organic Personality Syndrome
294.80 Atypical or Mixed Organic Brain Syndrome

Substance Use Disorders

Code in fifth digit: 1 = Continuous, 2 = Episodic, 3 = in Remission, 0 = Unspecified

305.0x Alcohol Abuse, _____
303.9x Alcohol Dependence (Alcoholism), _____
305.4x Barbiturate or similarly acting sedative or hypnotic Abuse, _____
304.1x Barbiturate or similarly acting sedative or hypnotic Dependence, _____
305.5x Opioid Abuse, _____
304.0x Opioid Dependence, _____
305.6x Cocaine Abuse, _____
305.7x Amphetamine or similarly acting sympathomimetic Abuse, _____
304.4x Amphetamine or similarly acting sympathomimetic Dependence, _____
305.9x Phencyclidine (PCP) or similarly acting arylcyclohexylamine Abuse, _____ (328.4x)
305.3x Hallucinogen Abuse, _____
305.2x Cannabis Abuse, _____
304.3x Cannabis Dependence, _____
305.1x Tobacco Dependence, _____
305.9x Other, mixed or unspecified Substance Abuse, _____
304.6x Other Specified Substance Dependence, _____
304.9x Unspecified Substance Dependence, _____
304.7x Dependence on Combination of Opioid and other Nonalcoholic Substance, _____
304.8x Dependence on Combination of Substances, excluding opioids and alcohol, _____

Schizophrenic Disorders

Code in fifth digit: 1 = Subchronic, 2 = Chronic, 3 = Subchronic with Acute Exacerbation, 4 = Chronic with Acute Exacerbation, 5 = in Remission, 0 = Unspecified.

SCHIZOPHRENIA

295.1x	Disorganized, _____
295.2x	Catatonic, _____
295.3x	Paranoid, _____
295.9x	Undifferentiated, _____
395.6x	Residual, _____

Paranoid Disorders

297.10	Paranoia
297.30	Shared Paranoid Disorder
298.30	Acute Paranoid Disorder
297.90	Atypical Paranoid Disorder

Psychotic Disorders Not Elsewhere Classified

295.40	Schizophreniform Disorder
298.80	Brief Reactive Psychosis
295.70	Schizoaffective Disorder
298.90	Atypical Psychosis

Neurotic Disorders

These are included in Affective, Anxiety, Somatoform, Dissociative, and Psychosexual Disorders. In order to facilitate the identification of the categories that in DSM-II were grouped together in the class of Neuroses, the DSM-II terms are included separately in parentheses after the corresponding categories. These DSM-II terms are included in ICD–9–CM and therefore are acceptable as alternatives to the recommended DSM-III terms that precede them.

Affective Disorders

Major Affective Disorders   Code Major Depressive Episode in fifth digit: 6 = in Remission, 4 = with Psychotic Features (the unofficial non-ICD–9–CM fifth digit 7 may be used instead to indicate that the psychotic features are mood-incongruent), 3 = with Melancholia, 2 = without Melancholia, 0 = Unspecified.

Code Manic Episode in fifth digit: 6 = in Remission, 4 = with Psychotic Features (the unofficial non-ICD–9–CM fifth digit 7 may be used instead to indicate that the psychotic features are mood-incongruent), 2 = without Psychotic Features, 0 = Unspecified.

BIPOLAR DISORDER

296.6x	Mixed, _____
296.4x	Manic, _____
296.5x	Depressed, _____

MAJOR DEPRESSION

296.2x	Single Episode, _____
296.3x	Recurrent, _____

Other Specific Affective Disorders

301.13	Cyclothymic Disorder
300.40	Dysthymic Disorder (or Depressive Neurosis)

Atypical Affective Disorders

296.70	Atypical Bipolar Disorder
296.82	Atypical Depression

Anxiety Disorders

PHOBIC DISORDERS (OR PHOBIC NEUROSES)

300.21	Agoraphobia with Panic Attacks
300.22	Agoraphobia without Panic Attacks
300.23	Social Phobia
300.29	Simple Phobia

ANXIETY STATES (OR ANXIETY NEUROSES)

300.01	Panic Disorder
300.02	Generalized Anxiety Disorder
300.30	Obsessive Compulsive Disorder (or Obsessive Compulsive Neurosis)

POST-TRAUMATIC STRESS DISORDER

308.30	Acute
309.81	Chronic or Delayed
300.00	Atypical Anxiety Disorder

Somatoform Disorders

300.81	Somatization Disorder
300.11	Conversion Disorder (or Hysterical Neurosis, Conversion Type)
307.80	Psychogenic Pain Disorder
300.70	Hypochondriasis (or Hypochondriacal Neurosis)
300.70	Atypical Somatoform Disorder (300.71)

Dissociative Disorders (or Hysterical Neuroses, Dissociative Type)

300.12	Psychogenic Amnesia
300.13	Psychogenic Fugue
300.14	Multiple Personality
300.60	Depersonalization Disorder (or Depersonalization Neurosis)
300.15	Atypical Dissociative Disorder

Psychosexual Disorders

Gender Identity Disorders   Indicate sexual history in the fifth digit of Transsexualism code: 1 = Asexual, 2 = Homosexual, 3 = Heterosexual, 0 = Unspecified

302.5x	Transsexualism, _____
302.60	Gender Identity Disorder of Childhood
302.85	Atypical Gender Identity Disorder

Paraphilias

302.81	Fetishism
302.30	Tranvestism
302.10	Zoophilia
302.20	Pedophilia
302.40	Exhibitionism
302.82	Voyeurism
302.83	Sexual Masochism
302.84	Sexual Sadism
302.90	Atypical Paraphilia

Psychosexual Dysfunctions

302.71	Inhibited Sexual Desire
302.72	Inhibited Sexual Excitement
302.73	Inhibited Female Orgasm
302.74	Inhibited Male Orgasm
302.75	Premature Ejaculation
302.76	Functional Dyspareunia
302.51	Functional Vaginismus
302.70	Atypical Psychosexual Dysfunction

Other Psychosexual Disorders

302.00	Ego-dystonic Homosexuality
302.89	Psychosexual Disorder not elsewhere classified

Factitious Disorders

300.16	Factitious Disorder with Psychological Symptoms
301.51	Chronic Factitious Disorder with Physical Symptoms
300.19	Atypical Factitious Disorder with Physical Symptoms

Disorders of Impulse Control Not Elsewhere Classified

312.31 Pathological Gambling
312.32 Kleptomania
312.33 Pyromania
312.34 Intermittent Explosive Disorder
312.35 Isolated Explosive Disorder
312.39 Atypical Impulse Control Disorder

Adjustment Disorder

309.00 with Depressed Mood
302.24 with Anxious Mood
309.28 with Mixed Emotional Features
309.30 with Disturbance of Conduct
309.40 with Mixed Disturbance of Emotions and Conduct
309.23 with Work (or Academic) Inhibition
309.83 with Withdrawal
309.90 with Atypical Features

Psychological Factors Affecting Physical Condition

Specify physical condition on Axis III.
316.00 Psychological Factors Affecting Physical Condition

PERSONALITY DISORDERS

Note: These are coded on Axis II.

301.00 Paranoid
301.20 Schizoid
301.22 Schizotypal
301.50 Histrionic
301.81 Narcissistic
301.70 Antisocial
301.83 Borderline
301.82 Avoidant
301.60 Dependent
301.40 Compulsive
301.84 Passive-Aggressive
301.89 Atypical, Mixed or other Personality Disorder

V Codes for Conditions Not Attributable to a Mental Disorder That Are a Focus of Attention or Treatment

V65.20 Malingering
V62.89 Borderline Intellectual Functioning (V62.88)
V71.01 Adult Antisocial Behavior
V71.02 Childhood or Adolescent Antisocial Behavior
V62.30 Academic Problem
V62.20 Occupational Problem
V62.82 Uncomplicated Bereavement
V15.81 Noncompliance with Medical Treatment
V62.89 Phase of Life Problem or Other Life Circumstance Problem
V61.10 Marital problem
V61.20 Parent-Child Problem
V61.80 Other Specified Family Circumstances
V62.81 Other Interpersonal Problem

Additional Codes

300.90 Unspecified Mental Disorder (Nonpsychotic)
V71.09 No Diagnosis or Condition on Axis I
799.90 Diagnosis or Condition Deferred on Axis I

V71.09 No Diagnosis on Axis II
799.90 Diagnosis Deferred on Axis II

AXIS III:
PHYSICAL DISORDERS OR CONDITIONS

Axis III permits the clinician to indicate any current physical disorder or condition that is potentially relevant to the understanding or management of the client. These are the conditions exclusive of the "mental disorders section" of ICD–9–CM. (The 9th edition of the International Classification of Diseases.) In some instances the condition may be etiologically significant; in other instances the physical disorder is important to the overall management of the client. In yet other instances, the clinician may wish to note the presence of other significant associated physical assessment findings, such as "soft neurological signs." Multiple diagnoses are permitted on this axis.

AXIS IV: SEVERITY OF PSYCHOSOCIAL STRESSORS

Code	Term	Adult Examples	Child or Adolescent Examples
1	None	No apparent psychosocial stressor	No apparent psychosocial stressor
2	Minimal	Minor violation of the law; small bank loan	Vacation with family
3	Mild	Argument with neighbor; change in work hours	Change in schoolteacher; new school year
4	Moderate	New career; death of close friend; pregnancy	Chronic parental fighting; change to new school; illness of close relative; birth of sibling
5	Severe	Serious illness in self or family; major financial loss; marital separation; birth of child	Death of peer; divorce of parents; arrest; hospitalization; persistent and harsh parental discipline
6	Extreme	Death of close relative; divorce	Death of parent or sibling; repeated physical or sexual abuse

AXIS IV—Continued			
Code	Term	Adult Examples	Child or Adolescent Examples
7	Cata–strophic	Concentration camp experience; devastating natural disaster	Multiple family deaths
0	Unspe–cified	No information, or not applicable	No information, or not applicable

AXIS V: HIGHEST LEVEL OF ADAPTIVE FUNCTIONING PAST YEAR

Levels	Adult Examples	Child or Adolescent Examples
1 SUPERIOR Unusually effective functioning in social relations, occupational functioning, and use of leisure time.	Single parent living in deteriorating neighborhood takes excellent care of children and home, has warm relations with friends, and finds time for pursuit of hobby.	A 12–year-old girl gets superior grades in school, is extremely popular among her peers, and excels in many sports. She does all of this with apparent ease and comfort.
2 VERY GOOD Better than average functioning in social relations, occupational functioning, and use of leisure time.	A 65–year-old retired widower does some volunteer work, often sees old friends, and pursues hobbies.	An adolescent boy gets excellent grades, works part-time, has several close friends, and plays banjo in a jazz band. He admits to some distress in "keeping up with everything."

AXIS V—Continued		
Levels	Adult Examples	Child or Adolescent Examples
3 GOOD No more than slight impairment in either social or occupational functioning.	A woman with many friends functions extremely well at a difficult job, but says "the strain is too much."	An 8–year-old boy does well in school, has several friends, but bullies younger children.
4 FAIR Moderate impairment in either social relations or occupational functioning, or some impairment in both.	A lawyer has trouble carrying through assignments; has several acquaintances, but hardly any close friends.	A 10–year-old girl does poorly in school, but has adequate peer and family relations.
5 POOR Marked impairment in either social relations or occupational functioning, or moderate impairment in both.	A man with one or two friends has trouble keeping a job for more than a few weeks.	A 14–year-old boy almost fails in school and has trouble getting along with his peers.
6 VERY POOR Marked impairment in both social relations and occupational functioning.	A woman is unable to do any of her housework and has violent outbursts toward family and neighbors.	A 6–year-old girl needs special help in all subjects and has virtually no peer relationships.
7 GROSSLY IMPAIRED Gross impairment in virtually all areas of functioning.	An elderly man needs supervision to maintain minimal personal hygiene and is usually incoherent.	A 4–year-old boy needs constant restraint to avoid hurting himself and is almost totally lacking in skills.
O UNSPECIFIED	No information.	No information.

NOTES

NOTES

NOTES